The Mild Traumatic Brain Injury WORKBOOK

Your Program for Regaining Cognitive Function & Overcoming Emotional Pain

DOUGLAS J. MASON, PSYD

New Harbinger Publications, Inc.

Publisher's Note

Distributed in Canada by Raincoast Books

Copyright © 2004 by Douglas J. Mason
New Harbinger Publications
5674 Shattuck Avenue
Oakland, CA 94609

This work is based on the ABC-123 Model of Neurocognitive Therapy. Copyright 2002 by Douglas J. Mason.

Information on pages 6-7 provided with permission from National Association of State Head Injury Administrators (2001). *Traumatic brain injury facts: emergency medical services*. Available from NASHIA, 4733 Bethesda Ave., Suite 330, Bethesda, MD 20816. www.nashia.org.

Cover design by Amy Shoup
Cover image by Digital Vision/Getty Images
Acquired by Spencer Smith
Text design by Tracy Marie Carlson

ISBN-10 1-57224-361-9
ISBN-13 978-1-57224-361-3

New Harbinger Publications' website address: www.newharbinger.com

17   16   15
15   14   13   12   11   10

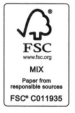
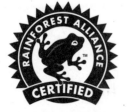

To my soul mate, Brenda: You make life's journey meaningful and fun. Thank you for being my partner, my love, and my friend and for sharing life's adventure.

To my beautiful daughters, Stephanie and Jenna, who teach me every day the value of innocence, wonderment, and continued curiosity.

Contents

Foreword · · · · · · · · · · · · · · · · ix

Acknowledgments · · · · · · · · · · · · · · · · xi

Introduction · · · · · · · · · · · · · · · · · 1
⌘ The Importance of Professional Help ⌘ Effort Is Essential ⌘ Exercise Your Mind, Heal Your Brain ⌘ One Step, One Day at a Time

CHAPTER 1
An Overview of MTB · · · · · · · · · · · · · 5
⌘ Warning Signs Related to Traumatic Brain Injury ⌘ Incidence of TBI ⌘ Symptoms of MTBI ⌘ Exercise: Gauging Your

Symptoms ⌘ Exercise: Symptom Checklist ⌘ Exercise: The Symptoms of PostConcussive Syndrome ⌘ Exercise: Letter Search

CHAPTER 2

Anatomy of the Brain · · · · · · · · · · · · · · · · · **15**
   ⌘ The five Cognitive Domains ⌘ Exercise: Cognitive Domains ⌘ Exercise: Maze 1
   ⌘ The Four Lobes ⌘ Important Brain Regions Related to Cognition ⌘ Exercise:
   Cognitive Domains

CHAPTER 3

What Happens to the Brain after an MTBI · · · · · · · · **25**
   ⌘ Types of MTBI ⌘ The Varieties of Damage in MTBI ⌘ How MTBI Affects Your
   Brain Function ⌘ Exercise: Maze 2

CHAPTER 4

Measuring the Severity of the Injury · · · · · · · · · · · **31**
   ⌘ Gauging Severity ⌘ When is Hospitalization Necessary? ⌘ Exercise: Symptom
   Severity Rating Scale ⌘ Exercise: Cognitive Anagrams ⌘ Exercise: Maze 3

CHAPTER 5

Setting Goals · **37**
   ⌘ Exercise: Maze 4 ⌘ Set Goals for yourself ⌘ Exercise: Establishing Goals
   ⌘ Use Your Goals as a Guide ⌘ Exercise: Number Search

CHAPTER 6

Managing Your Medical Care · · · · · · · · · · · · · · **43**
   ⌘ Choose One Primary-care Physician ⌘ Exercise: Maze 5 ⌘ Your Neurocognitive
   Rehabilitation Team ⌘ The Neurological Evaluation

CHAPTER 7

Physical Aspects of Traumatic Brain Injury · · · · · · · **51**
   ⌘ Exercise: Symbol Search ⌘ Headaches ⌘ Weakness ⌘ Poor Balance
   ⌘ Seizures ⌘ Sexuality ⌘ Fatigue ⌘ Exercise ⌘ Moving toward Rehabilitation

CHAPTER 8

The Senses · **59**
   ⌘ The Complexity of the Senses ⌘ Exercise: Maze 6 ⌘ Exercise: Testing Your
   Cranial Nerves

CHAPTER 9

Attention · 67

⌘ Review of Maze Exercises   ⌘ Take a Look   ⌘ Tuning in to Attention
⌘ Exercise: Selective Attention   ⌘ Exercise: Alternating Attention   ⌘ Exercise:
Divided Attention   ⌘ Improving Your Attention   ⌘ Exercise: Active Attention Vs.
Passive Attention, Part One   ⌘ Exercise: Active Attention Vs. Passive Attention, Part
Two   ⌘ Review the Attention Exercises   ⌘ Taking it to the Outside World

CHAPTER 10

Memory · 81

⌘ An Overview of Memory   ⌘ The Left Brain or the Right Brain?   ⌘ Exercise: Visual
or Verbal Memory Orientation   ⌘ Building Memory Muscle   ⌘ Exercise: Cleaning the
Attic   ⌘ Exercise: Cleaning the Attic—Free Recall vs. Recogntion   ⌘ Exercise: Talking
to Remember   ⌘ A Word on Relaxation   ⌘ Additional Help

CHAPTER 11   by: Teri DeFrano, MS, CCC-SLP

Cognitive Communication · 97

⌘ Language and Cognition   ⌘ Exercise: Verbal Association   ⌘ Recovering Your
Language Abilities   ⌘ Exercise: Word Puzzles   ⌘ Exercise: Purposeful Pronunciation
and Compulsory Comprehension   ⌘ Language in Your Life

CHAPTER 12   with Susie Rentz

Visuospatial Processing · 107

⌘ The Way that Vision Works   ⌘ Exercise: Block Decipher   ⌘ Exercise: Visual
Discrimination   ⌘ Repairing Your VisuoSpatial Deficits   ⌘ Exercise: Locate the Regions
of the Brain   ⌘ Exercise: Figure Ground   ⌘ Your Sight, Your World

CHAPTER 13

Depression · 119

⌘ Depression and MTBI are Intertwined   ⌘ Exercise: Depression Assessment
⌘ The Problem of Depression and MTBI   ⌘ Exercise: The Downward Arrow
⌘ Seeking Professional Help   ⌘ A Word of Reassurance

CHAPTER 14

Anxiety · 129

⌘ The Nature of Anxiety   ⌘ Anxiety and MTBI   ⌘ Relaxation   ⌘ Exercise:
Learning to Relax   ⌘ Exercise: Progressive Muscle Relaxation   ⌘ Exercise: Abdominal
Breathing   ⌘ Exercise: Guided Visualization   ⌘ Relaxation Every day

CONCLUSION

Putting It All Together · · · · · · · · · · · · **139**

Goals Review   ⌘   Exercise: Goals Review   ⌘   In Closing

APPENDIX A

Glossary/Pronunciation and Comprehension Answer Key · · · · · · · · · **143**

APPENDIX B

Resources · **147**

APPENDIX C

Answers to Exercises and Puzzles · · · · · · · · · · · **153**

Chapter 1   ⌘   Exercise: Letter Search Answers
Chapter 2   ⌘   Exercise: Maze 1 Answer
Chapter 3   ⌘   Exercise: Maze 2 Answer
Chapter 4   ⌘   Exercise: Cognitive Anagrams Answers   ⌘   Exercise: Maze 3 Answer
Chapter 5   ⌘   Exercise: Maze 4 Answers   ⌘   Exericse: Number Search Answers
Chapter 6   ⌘   Exercise: Maze 5 Answers
Chapter 7   ⌘   Exercise: Symbol Search Answers
Chapter 8   ⌘   Exercise: Maze 6 Answers
Chapter 10   ⌘   Exercise: Attic Cleaning Answers
Chapter 11   ⌘   Exercise: Verbal Associations Answers   ⌘   Exercise: Word Puzzles
                    Answers
Chapter 12   ⌘   Exercise: Block Decipher Answers   ⌘   Exercise: Visual Discrimination
                    Answers   ⌘   Exercise: Locate the Regions of the Brain
              ⌘   Exercise: Figure Ground Answers

References · **173**

Foreword

I have been evaluating and treating patients with mild traumatic brain injury for the last twenty years. Under my supervision, they have undergone testing (CT scans, MRIs, EEGs, PET scans, and SPECT scans), therapy (physical and psychological), medication management (with antidepressants, anticonvulsants, stimulants, and cognitive enhancers) and subspecialty consultations (with neuropsychologists, ophthalmologists, and otolaryngologists). Despite this, many reported ongoing problems with concentration, orientation, language, mood, judgment, attention and memory.

I became aware of *The Mild Traumatic Brain Injury Workbook* several years ago and began recommending it to my MTBI patients. I have had hundreds use the workbook and see improvement in the areas just mentioned.

In our current cost-conscious environment, I have found that by having my patients use the workbook, I can reduce the amount of testing, therapy, medications, and consultations that are needed as patients get better through their own efforts.

The Mild Traumatic Brain Injury Workbook allows patients to regain their self-esteem, since they are in control of their recovery.

I anticipate that you, too, will find this workbook helpful in improving the quality of your life.

—Marc Irwin Sharfman, MD, director of the Headache and Neurological Treatment Institute
in Longwood, FL, and volunteer faculty, assistant professor of neurology in the Department
of Neurology and the University of Central Florida College of Medicine

Acknowledgments

First of all I would like to extend my gratitude to Mr. Spencer Smith. Without his kind assistance, expertise and dedication this work would not have been possible. I would also like to thank all of my patients who have taught me the meaning of courage and the strength of endurance. I would like to thank my beautiful wife Brenda for years of dedication and friendship and in assisting in this long project.

Introduction

Because you picked up this book, we can assume that you or a family member has undergone one of the most challenging medical injuries existing—mild traumatic brain injury, or MTBI. MTBI is a cluster of psychological and emotional difficulties that occur when a person has had severe trauma to the head. It is a curable condition, but many people live with these types of injuries without any medical guidance or psychological assistance. *The Mild Traumatic Brain Injury Workbook* represents a multistep approach to addressing your injuries. Throughout the book I will provide you with education on head injuries and information about what you might expect while navigating your course of recovery. This book will guide you through the process of examining where your deficits may be and help you to determine to what degree these deficits may affect you. I will give you the tools to better understand how the injury impacts your life and how to deal with this impact.

The exercises within this book serve many purposes. They will help you to quantify the level of damage you've experienced and identify your strengths. The exercises have been tested by more than a hundred patients with different levels of brain injury and are designed to examine and treat very specific regions of the brain. With the information we gain from the exercises, you can compare your performance with that of others and determine your level of impairment. Therefore, the process of recovery will coincide with identifying and addressing your symptoms. As you progress through the book and complete the exercises, I will guide you in examining and quantifying different aspects of your *cognitive function* (the operation of your mind and thoughts).

Your recovery process will not only include the cognitive aspects of healing—those related to thinking—but will also encompass the emotional influences, social impacts, professional consequences, and economic hardships that you may encounter. This recovery process will initially entail some retraining of cognitive functions like attention, emotions, and memory. We will also explore strategies that will help you compensate for your specific identified deficits and begin to rebuild cognitive function. We will set and achieve realistic goals that will guide your recovery.

Keep in mind that this book shouldn't take the place of your physician's advice or the advice of other qualified medical experts. After sustaining a head injury, the first step is always to get a comprehensive medical and neurological (nervous system) examination. To assist you with this, I provide a section in the book on what to expect during a neurological workup and how to better communicate your concerns to your physician. You should also follow up on an outpatient basis at least once to ensure that no additional damage or symptoms are developing. Appendix B can guide you on how to obtain any needed resources. The brain, like any other part of the body, can swell when damaged, which can greatly affect the blood flow and thus the availability of oxygen. As you will soon see, the damage from a mild head injury can be subtle, and it often requires a period of weeks to months to fully appreciate the impact of these subtle changes. Remember, this book is intended as a source of education and as one of many resources to assist you in the healing process. This workbook will best assist you in this process only after the essential initial medical evaluations have taken place.

THE IMPORTANCE OF PROFESSIONAL HELP

This book is intended for those who have noticed changes in their memory or other cognitive functioning as a result of a closed head injury (that is, one in which the skull is not penetrated). It is not intended for those who have a debilitating neurological disorder that impairs daily functioning. Although we will cover many of the techniques that are utilized with severe cognitive impairment, attempting to self-administer these techniques without the assistance of a qualified therapist may be counterproductive and possibly damaging. If you believe that you have cognitive impairment that severely impacts your day-to-day life, it's essential that you undergo a comprehensive neurological evaluation. Diagnosing cognitive impairments is complex and well beyond the scope of this book. A medical professional is better equipped to conduct a comprehensive evaluation that can help you in getting the assistance that you might need. Most people find that a certain level of comfort is usually found from consulting a medical professional, no matter what the diagnosis or prognosis. Many cognitive problems can be treated effectively, so don't be afraid to ask for help.

EFFORT IS ESSENTIAL

This book provides exercises designed to identify and treat memory problems and other cognitive difficulties that you might be experiencing as a result of your head injury. A primary goal is to help you to identify and use your existing strengths. Each exercise builds upon the previous one and serves to enhance upcoming lessons. The benefits that you derive from this book will be directly proportional to your commitment to reading the material in order and participating in each exercise. Proceed with enthusiasm and determination, and you will reap the maximum benefit. Effort, an open mind, and commitment are essential in your recovery from your head injury. It will seem at times that some of the exercises are randomly scattered throughout the book, but it's important that you complete each exercise in order, as they will be reviewed later to help you to determine where your strengths and deficits lie.

EXERCISE YOUR MIND, HEAL YOUR BRAIN

We are learning more and more about how the brain is able to reroute, repair, and even regenerate neurons and neural pathways. It has even been shown that the *hippocampus* (the primary memory center of the brain) has some capacity for the regrowth of neurons. This *plasticity* (ability to self-heal) of the brain is greatly enhanced through activity and by the proper application of exercise. This approach to what's called neurocognitive rehabilitation is a "top-down" approach where the workings of the mind are viewed like a muscle. By exercising the larger muscle groups, the smaller groups will inherently become strengthened.

Your brain is adaptive and pliable, and it can be reshaped and rebuilt, but this process takes some education, effort, and energy. This energy must be continuously and strategically applied for the "muscle" to grow, thrive, and flourish. In completing the exercises, you will be guided in tailoring this program to fit your personal style. I will help you not only in sculpting and shaping your thinking and cognitive abilities and in applying these learned skills to your everyday life, but also in maintaining your healthy memory and cognitive functioning.

ONE STEP, ONE DAY AT A TIME

This book is intended to be read in the order presented. Although some of you may want to read only the portions that most apply to you, I recommend that you dive in and read it all. This is because many of the skills are hierarchically based, going from one important gradient to the next, with each new task building upon previously learned skills. There will be times when it's necessary to take a break and work in a specific area before progressing any further. This is fine, and I encourage you to proceed at your own pace.

Pay special attention to words or concepts that are italicized throughout the text, as these are key concepts and terms. When something is italicized, it is being introduced for the first time and a definition will follow. It's important that you slow down your reading when you come across these introductions and be sure that you understand the concept being introduced.

As a caveat to my point that effort is essential, good effort is respectful of limits. There is a limit to how much new information the mind can absorb in one sitting, and this limit should be respected. Retention of information is better facilitated through exposure to the information in small chunks over a sustained period of time. In other words, many small readings will be more beneficial than one or two cram sessions. Therefore I recommend that you not read more than you're able retain during any one sitting. When you find that you're fatigued and having difficulty focusing or comprehending what you read, it is time to put the book down and rest.

There are exercises throughout this book. These exercises have a multitude of functions. In some cases they are provided as a simple mental workout that will help to keep you sharp and aware as you proceed through your recovery process. This is particularly true for the exercises that are in the early parts of the book.

As you progress, you will find that the exercises are directed more and more toward specific parts of your cognitive function. There are exercises that give you quantitative assessments of particular processes in your mind and others that will start to help you repair the parts of your mind that have been damaged.

Please work through each of the exercises. Try to have fun with them! They will help you in many ways. If you are incapable of completing the exercises given in this book, then your problem is more severe than we can handle here. If it turns out you are having a problem in this regard, I would suggest that you speak to your general care physician immediately.

Now that we have covered the basics of the workbook, we can move to chapter 1, where we'll begin to look at some of the dynamics associated with MTBI.

CHAPTER 1

An Overview of MTBI

A traumatic brain injury (TBI) is damage to the brain due to externally inflicted trauma. Mild traumatic brain injury (MTBI) is simply the lower-grade forms of TBI. In this book we will be focusing on brain injuries that are considered mild, but first let's look at TBI in general. This type of injury is caused by a penetrating or blunt trauma or from the force of rapid acceleration and deceleration. The initial results of a TBI include neurological or neuropsychological damage, skull fracture, amnesia, impaired consciousness or unconsciousness, brain lesions, or even death (Thurman et al. 1994). *Neurological damage* refers broadly to injury to the nervous system, especially the brain. *Neuropsychological damage* is injury to the nervous system as it relates to your thoughts and feelings. A TBI is one of the most devastating events that a person can endure, and the ramifications can be equally devastating to the afflicted individual's family. The long-term effects continue to be the subject of much debate, research, and controversy. The functional outcome and emotional consequences associated with TBI are complex and tend to be unique to each individual. Traditional rehabilitation efforts often show limited success, with results that are mixed at best. This is even true for head injuries that are classified as mild.

Medical treatment is always essential in the event of a TBI. There are many signs and symptoms that may indicate an immediate need for medical assistance. We'll start this chapter off by identifying some of the warning signs following a head injury. If you or a loved one is experiencing any of these symptoms, then the appropriate medical contacts should be made. The following is reproduced with the kind permission of the National Association of State Head Injury Administrators (2001). (See Resources.)

WARNING SIGNS RELATED TO TRAUMATIC BRAIN INJURY

Following a brain injury or concussion, presence of the following symptoms should be monitored. These symptoms may not present themselves until days or weeks after the injury (National Association of State Head Injury Administrators (2001). *Traumatic brain injury facts: emergency medical services.* Available from NASHIA, 4733 Bethesda Ave., Suite 330, Bethesda, MD 20816. www.nashia.org).

A child should be taken to the ER, see his/her physician, or call 911 immediately if he/she:

- can not be awakened (call 911)

- remains increasingly sleepy

- can not stop throwing up

- has a seizure, sudden onset of dreaming, or a continued fixed stare

- has dramatic mood swings or remains agitated or sad

- has problems seeing or has blurred or double vision

- seems incoherent, disoriented, or confused or has difficulty speaking

- has blood or clear fluid coming from the ears or nose

- has continued headaches or neck or back stiffness

- has pupils (black portion of eyes) that are different sizes

- has problems walking, with balance or dizziness

An adult should be taken to the ER, see his/her physician, or call 911 if he/she:

- has trouble answering simple questions, seems disoriented, or is unable to recognize friends, family, or surroundings

- has difficulty waking up or seems groggy all the time

- continues to experience headaches, especially if they continue after medication is taken

- has dramatic changes in personality or in emotions

- continues to throw up eight hours after the injury or starts to throw up one to two hours after the injury

- has pupils that are different sizes

- has difficulty walking or with balance

- has double vision, blurred vision, or blind spots in vision

- has difficulty talking, slurred speech, speech that does not make sense, or continues to ask the same questions

- has seizures or convulsions, daydreams constantly, or has fixed stares

- has blood or clear fluid coming from the nose or ears

If symptoms are getting worse or if you can answer yes to any of the following questions, you should seek medical treatment:

- Does he/she get lost or seem confused?

- Has there been a dramatic personality change or does he/she seem angry all of the time?

- Does he/she have more difficulty making decisions?

- Are there noticeable problems in thinking (poor memory, poor attention or concentration, difficulty in learning, speaking, or understanding)?

- Is there a significant drop in work, school, or social performance or activities?

INCIDENCE OF TBI

Every year in the United States as many as two million people sustain a head injury that results in cognitive complications requiring treatment. One in forty of these sustain brain injuries that result in lifelong, debilitating impairment (Chestnut, Carney, and Maynard 1999). Prevalence is estimated at 3.5 million to 6.5 million men, women, and children who are currently living with the long-term consequences of a TBI. The majority of TBIs occur as a result of auto accidents, while interpersonal violence, falls, and recreational injuries make up most of the other incidents. According to the Centers for Disease Control (2001), 75 percent of all TBI's are considered mild in nature. However, traumatic brain injury is responsible for approximately 50,000 deaths every year, and is twice as likely to ocur in men as women. It is the leading cause of death in children and young adults. The highest incidence is among persons aged fifteen to twenty-four years and seventy-five years or older. Alcohol is reported to be involved in over half of all TBIs (Centers for Disease Control and Prevention 2001).

SYMPTOMS OF MTBI

There are many symptoms associated with MTBI that can affect all aspects of your functioning. Below is a summary of the more common symptoms broken down into type of function. Next to each symptom is a box. As you review the symptoms, place an "x" in the boxes that apply to you and reflect symptoms that you are currently experiencing. We'll be using the little lines in front of the boxes next.

EXERCISE: GAUGING YOUR SYMPTOMS

Emotional

____   ☐ Depression

____   ☐ Anxiety

____   ☐ Hopelessness

____   ☐ Helplessness

____   ☐ Reduced confidence

____   ☐ Apathy (lack of drive or initiative)

____   ☐ Irritability

____   ☐ Emotional numbness

____   ☐ Intense fear

Behavioral

____   ☐ Impatience

____   ☐ Anger

____   ☐ Frustration

____   ☐ Confrontational behaviors

____   ☐ Impulsivity

____   ☐ Increased avoidance of situations or activities that feel uncomfortable (like being around others, riding in cars)

____   ☐ Withdrawal

Physical

____   ☐ Headaches

____   ☐ Chronic pain

____   ☐ Fatigue

____ ☐ Weakness or numbness

____ ☐ Changes in vision

____ ☐ Changes in hearing

____ ☐ Other sensory changes (touch, taste, smell)

____ ☐ Changes in sleep

____ ☐ Changes in appetite

____ ☐ Vertigo (dizziness)

____ ☐ Nausea

____ ☐ Impairments in fine motor speed and coordination

____ ☐ Changes in sexual functioning

Cognitive

____ ☐ Changes in attention

____ ☐ Diminished memory

____ ☐ Slowed speed of mental processing

____ ☐ Confusion

____ ☐ Disorientation

____ ☐ Changes in decision making

____ ☐ Alterations in judgment

____ ☐ Changes in ability to plan and organize

____ ☐ Changes in visual processing (difficulty in judging distance, spatial relations)

____ ☐ Difficulties with language comprehension or production

____ ☐ Increased distractibility

Social

____ ☐ Changes in relationships

____ ☐ Changed ability to engage in hobbies and leisure activities

_____ ☐ Decreased ability to perform at work or school

_____ ☐ Isolation

_____ ☐ Increased alienation from others

A word of encouragement: most people see significant improvement in these symptoms within the first six months after sustaining the injury. For others, the healing process lasts up to a year or longer.

EXERCISE: SYMPTOM CHECKLIST

Go back and review all of the symptoms that you checked in the preceding exercise. After you have checked all of the items that apply to you, the next step is to prioritize each of these symptoms according to their level of severity. On the line next to each box that is checked, rate the symptom on a scale from one to five. One is the least severe and five is the most severe. Here's another way to look at it:

1 = marginal symptoms (I notice a small difference, but it rarely affects my life.)

2 = mild symptoms (I notice some difference, but it only occasionally gets in the way of my daily functioning.)

3 = moderate symptoms (There is a definite difference, and it affects me to a significant degree on a daily basis.)

4 = severe symptoms (There is a profound difference and it almost always prevents me from functioning the way that I used to.)

5 = debilitating symptoms (There is such an impairment that I am unable to function.)

Go through all of the checked symptoms and rate them now.

Now let's take this a step further. In the following space provided, list each of the symptoms that you checked in the order of how much the symptom is influencing your life. Number one should be the most severe symptom (the highest number assigned) and the last one on your list should be the least severe. In cases where you have several symptoms rated with the same number, make a subjective decision as to the severity of each symptom.

1. _____

2. _____

3. _____

4. _____

5. _____

6. _____

7. _____

8. _____

9. _____

10. _____

11. _____

12. _____

13. _____

14. _____

15. _____

16. _____

17. _____

18. _____

19. _____

20. _____

21. _____

22. _____

23. _____

24. _____

25. _____

Postconcussive Syndrome

Postconcussive syndrome is a group of symptoms that often result from an MTBI. Many, if not most, mild to moderate head injuries result in postconcussive syndrome. Symptoms associated with the syndrome are often subtle and frequently go undiagnosed. Check the symptoms below that you experience. They are similar to the ones in the last exercise, but it's important to assess them again here. If you have ten or more symptoms below, then you are probably experiencing postconcussive syndrome, and a thorough medical and/or neurological exam is necessary.

EXERCISE: THE SYMPTOMS OF POSTCONCUSSIVE SYNDROME

☐ Memory impairment

☐ Alterations in attention

☐ Disturbances in mood

☐ Headaches

☐ Fatigue (lack of endurance)

☐ Difficulties with organization

☐ Limitations in abstract thinking

☐ Lack of initiative (apathy)

☐ Lack of inhibition

☐ Slowed thinking or information processing

☐ Sensory and perceptual disturbances

☐ Dizziness (difficulties with balance)

☐ Sexual inhibition or lack of inhibition

☐ Sleep impairments

☐ Problems with language production or comprehension

☐ Visual disturbances (blurred or double vision)

☐ Reduced concentration

☐ Increased sensitivity to noise or light

☐ Chronic pain, numbness, or weakness

☐ Changes in mood (anxiety or depression)

☐ Irritability

The lists in these exercises will serve as your guide to your healing process. Different portions of the book will address ways to treat and compensate for these symptoms.

There are many people who, after sustaining a head injury, receive a variety of tests—including imaging tests that provide a look inside the skull and other neurological and neuropsychological tests—and are found to have limited or no deficits. These individuals are often told that they are normal and "lucky" and that they should continue to go about their normal routine. But sometimes these people begin to notice significant changes in their cognitive and emotional functioning once they get back to work or school. They find that they feel sad, tire easily, and have difficulty concentrating. They may have difficulty with calculations or in finding words that normally come to them easily. Along with the physical healing process, there is a natural cognitive and emotional healing process. In the following pages I'll guide you through that process. You'll have the current medical information to help you navigate through these challenges, and exercises to assist you in determining where your deficits lie and in fine-tuning the cognitive functions that have been damaged. You'll also learn compensatory strategies to help you in your recovery.

But before we move on, let's do a simple letter search. This game will help you to fine-tune your attention. Later in the book you'll use these results to diagnose where some of your cognitive deficits may lie. These search puzzles can be slow going, but don't get discouraged.

EXERCISE: LETTER SEARCH

Complete the letter search below. Letter sequences go in all directions, including backward and diagonally. Time yourself and write below the number of minutes that it took you to complete it below. Check your answers in appendix C when finished.

A	B	G	I	C	E	A	B	A	B	H	J	D	B	G
J	A	D	F	J	B	C	H	G	A	A	I	F	D	I
D	F	F	C	C	B	E	D	C	F	H	A	D	E	G
B	H	A	F	I	C	H	A	D	C	F	J	B	F	D
A	F	J	J	E	H	I	B	F	G	D	C	H	A	F
B	D	G	I	E	C	A	A	J	C	H	D	B	J	F
C	D	G	F	J	D	H	A	D	F	A	A	G	H	C
E	A	E	I	G	D	E	B	G	G	F	C	J	B	G
C	F	H	C	A	B	G	D	D	G	G	B	C	B	A
G	B	D	I	G	C	J	D	C	G	C	I	J	A	E
I	B	D	E	C	B	B	A	F	G	F	D	I	J	B
B	E	I	B	A	A	B	C	H	A	I	A	A	A	I
B	E	H	H	B	E	E	I	B	G	J	I	D	I	C
A	F	D	H	J	I	J	A	A	D	A	I	B	E	H
D	A	G	E	C	I	C	B	C	G	E	I	H	G	B

ABGIC	JAFDG	DHADF	IAHEG	IEEBH	CFIJA
DCFHA	CFHCA	CBJHF	DFAJI	DEFAJ	CIEBH
CIADG	GEIAJ	AJIJH	IEABC	CAIGD	DGFBI
BAFCG	ABIEB	CABHF	DFHBC	ABCBG	ACEHI
BHAFI	DGADH	CIEEJ	CHAIA	CECGI	GCIJA

Time: _____ minutes

CHAPTER 2

Anatomy of the Brain

In this chapter we will begin to learn about the complex functions of the brain. Traumatic brain injury can affect the brain in many ways. Both the degree of injury and the location of the injury greatly influence the outcome and impairment. Learning about the brain's functions will help us to later understand what happens to the brain as a result of an MTBI. First we will divide the brain's functioning into five categories or domains. The cognitive domains are:

- Memory

- Executive functioning (for instance, planning, decision making, impulse control)

- Attention

- Language and communication

- Sensory and motor functions (visuospatial processing)

The location of some of the functions of these domains is depicted below.

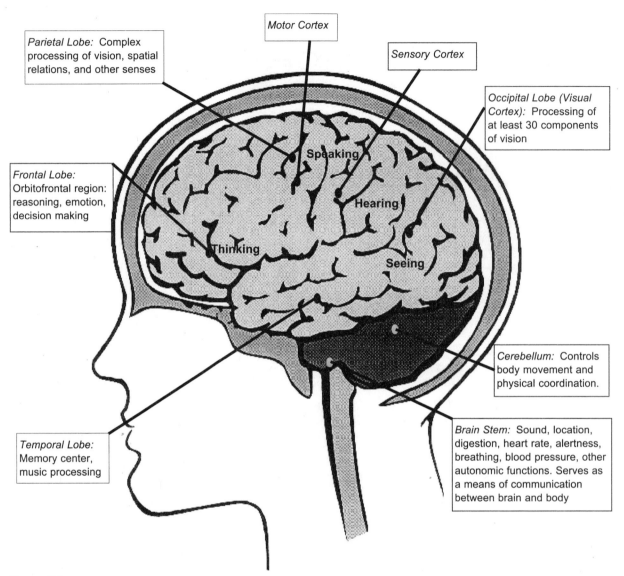

Figure 2.1

THE FIVE COGNITIVE DOMAINS

It's time to go into more detail about the five cognitive domains listed on the previous page. Remember that this is just an overview. Later in the book, I will be addressing most of these in much greater detail and will give you exercises that are designed to help you regain function in each of these domains.

Memory

Memory is a primary function that is often affected by MTBI. Memory disorders interfere with numerous processes, including new learning and relearning, recall, recognition, and rote memory. Memory disorders frequently trigger apathy about learning and are often caused by acquired deficits in attention. We will cover memory in much greater detail in subsequent chapters.

Executive Functioning

Executive functioning covers a wide variety of skills. These are the skills that the successful "executive" has to master, like time management, judgment, and planning. That's why these operations are referred to as "executive functions." These functions are controlled by the front of the brain. Given the physical location of the frontal lobes, executive skills are almost always affected to some degree by an MTBI. Another consideration is the wiring of the brain. Many *subcortical* (lower brain) regions are wired to *cortical* areas (higher areas of the brain) through the frontal lobes. Damage to the frontal lobes therefore affects not only the functions that are governed by the frontal lobes, but also the connections of other brain regions that run through this area. The frontal lobes govern a wide variety of functions, including awareness, insight, judgment, cognitive flexibility, rage, apathy, attention, fine motor initiation, planning, and behaviors. Impairment in executive function is beyond the scope of this book and should be addressed by professionals trained in these areas. For this reason it will not be addressed in the cognitive impairment portion of the book.

Attention

Attention is the foundation for all the other cognitive domains. It is essentially your ability to donate a given amount of cognitive energy in order to perform the task at hand. It allows you to organize tasks into a coherent, logical pattern that makes them easier to accomplish. If executive function is named thus because of its ability to help you perform executive-type tasks, attention would be a governor—directing your cognitive resources to where they need to be at any given time. Attention is finite, as it has a limited capacity. This capacity is controlled by both arousal (how aroused or stirred up we are) and velocity (how fast we can mentally process information). Impairments in attention are among the most common symptoms associated with acquired brain damage, and because the attention system is the foundation of other cognitive processes, the ramifications of attentional deficits seem all encompassing. Fortunately, research has demonstrated that attentional deficits are often responsive to neurocognitive therapy (Sohlberg and Mateer 1987).

Language and Communication

Language and communication disorders result from two types of dysfunction—aphasia and dysarthria. *Aphasia,* the loss of the ability to understand words, results from damage to the receptive and expressive centers in the frontal, parietal, occipital, and temporal lobes of the cerebral cortex. Information processing, verbal expression, and language interpretation are disrupted when injury to these parts of the brain occurs. *Dysarthria* is impaired neuromuscular control of the facial, oral, and laryngeal muscles needed for speech articulation. Researchers report overall good recovery of basic language skills with treatment, but deficits in analysis and expressive language skills (ability to talk) continue beyond one year after injury.

Sensory and Motor Functions

The senses are the first step in thinking (cognition). They are our link to the outside world and allow us to monitor and process the data in the environment around us. For the most part, motor functions will only be covered in this book as they relate to the other cognitive domains (like the motor functions of speech). Motor impairments secondary to MTBI require the assistance of a professional physical therapist. The primary sensory system that we will focus on in this book is the visual system. Within the visual system we will identify two primary systems: the spatial system, which answers the question of where something is and the visual form system, which answers the questions of what something is. These systems will be addressed later in detail.

EXERCISE: COGNITIVE DOMAINS

List the five cognitive domains below:

1. _____

2. _____

3. _____

4. _____

5. _____

Whether you remembered one or all five of the cognitive domains without referring back to the section, let's anchor that knowledge a little deeper into your memory. Let's take the first letter of each word and create an acronym. This *mnemonic* (memory technique) is called "acronym association." The acronym now represents the data to be remembered.

Memory

Executive functioning

Attention

Language

Sensorimotor functioning

The acronym is MEALS. With the MEALS acronym you now only have one piece of information to remember. Once you recall that one piece (the acronym), you'll be triggered to remember all five pieces of information the acronym represents.

There will be several maze exercises scattered throughout the next several chapters of the book. Please complete each one as you come to it. We will be coming back to these exercises in the cognitive rehabilitation portion of the book.

EXERCISE: MAZE 1

Using a pencil, start in the lower left corner of the maze and find your way to the finish in the upper right corner. Time yourself while you complete the following maze. Write down your time in seconds below the maze. In the next few chapters we will do several of these and then later review them as a way to determine how well your attention and visual scanning are functioning. You can compare your solution to the one in appendix C.

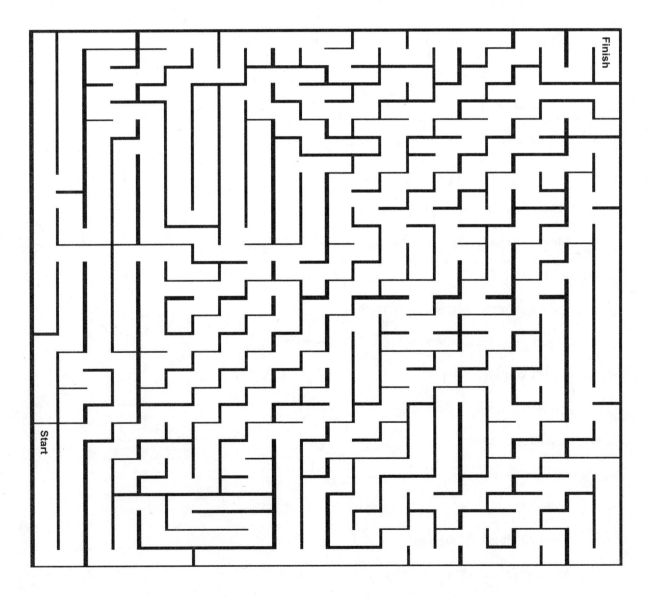

Time: _____ seconds

Now that we've looked at some of the functions of the brain, let's move on to the anatomy.

THE FOUR LOBES

Referring back to figure 2.1, let's now examine the different locations where various brain functions are located. The brain can be broken down into four main lobes. Starting in the front and moving clockwise, these are the frontal, parietal, occipital, and temporal lobes. The lists below describe the functions within each lobe.

The frontal lobe controls

- Initiation and inhibition of behaviors

- Decision making and problem solving (executive functions)

- Level of awareness and motivation

- Language expression

- Judgment and social behaviors

- Some emotions

- Attention and concentration

- Movement and integration of motor functions with other senses

The parietal lobe controls

- Tactile perception and sense of touch

- Processing of spatial information

The occipital lobe controls

- Visual input and perception

- Reading perception

The temporal lobe controls

- Memory

- Comprehension of language

- Music appreciation

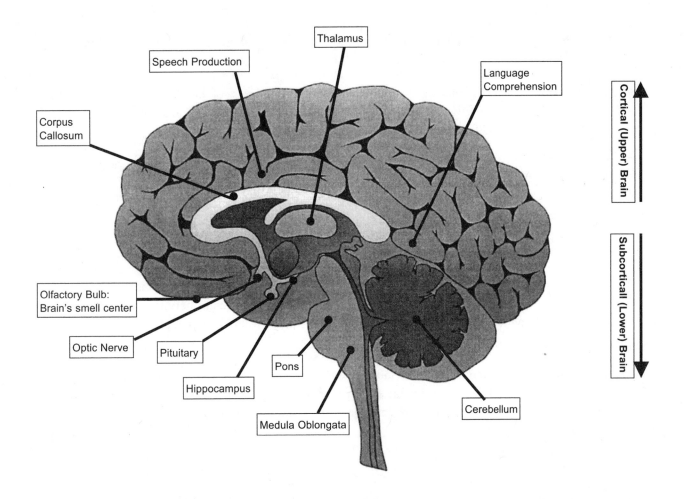

Figure 2.2

IMPORTANT BRAIN REGIONS RELATED TO COGNITION

This portion of the book is technical in nature and is intended for those more interested in the structures of the brain. You can also use it as a future reference if you find that you need to look up specific information on areas of the brain.

- **Amygdala:** Responsible for emotional integration of sensory input and memories.

- **Basal ganglia:** Located deep in the hemispheres. The basal ganglia are made up of the globus pallidus, caudate nucleus, and amygdala. Forms a circuit with the cortex. Important in the regulation of movement and in habit learning. Works closely with the frontal lobes.

- **Brain stem:** Connection from the spinal cord to lower areas of the brain. Responsible for autonomic functions such as heart rate, blood pressure, and the like. Motor and sensory neurons pass through the brain stem.

- **Broca's area:** Located in the left frontal lobe. Involved in the production of fluent speech.

- **Caudate nucleus:** Part of the neostriatum, which is part of basal ganglia. Receives projections from the neocortex and connects through the putamen and globus pallidus to the thalamus and finally to the motor area of the cortex.

- **Cerebellum:** The back portion of the brain that assists in coordinating movement. Damage often results in *ataxia* (uncoordinated voluntary muscle movements).

- **Cerebrum:** The largest part of the brain, divided into the left and right cerebral hemispheres. These upper portions of the brain are believed to be predominantly responsible for higher-order functions. Divided into the left and right cerebral hemispheres.

- **Left cerebral hemisphere:** In most people the left cerebral hemisphere is responsible for speech, math, reading, and writing. Damage to the left hemisphere often results in problems with verbal communication and problems with movement on the right side of the body.

- **Right cerebral hemisphere:** In most people the right cerebral hemisphere is responsible for visuospatial skills, direction, attention, and the regulation of emotions. Damage to this area will affect movement on the left side of the body and visuospatial abilities.

- **Corpus callosum:** Connects the two hemispheres of the brain, allowing for communication between them.

- **Frontal lobes:** Responsible for higher-order functioning (judgment, abstraction, and motivation) and the production of speech and has influence on personality. Damage results in difficulty with verbal expression, difficulty concentrating, and lack of emotional control. In the back of the frontal lobes are the motor areas that control voluntary movements. Damage results in *contralateral paralysis*, or paralysis on the opposite side of the body.

- **Hippocampus:** Structure in the brain believed to be responsible for the processing and coordination of memory functioning. It is the end point of the cortex and the ultimate destination of multiple cortical and subcortical processes.

- **Neurons:** Cells in the brain that store and process information.

- **Neurotransmitters:** Chemicals produced by the neurons that carry information from neuron to neuron. Specific neurotransmitters are responsible for specific tasks (for instance, dopamine is responsible for movement).

- **Occipital lobes:** Located in the back of the brain. Responsible for regulation and processing of sight.

- **Parietal lobes:** The *anterior* (front part) of the parietal lobes is responsible for tactile discrimination and recognition. The *posterior* (back part) of the parietal lobe is responsible for attention. The left parietal lobe is responsible for reading, writing, arithmetic, and performance of learned information. Its other function is speech. The right parietal lobe is responsible for the comprehension of visuospatial relationships and understanding facial expressions and tones in speech.

■ **Substantia nigra:** Connects basal ganglia to the midbrain. Provides dopamine to the basal ganglia.

■ **Temporal lobes:** Important for memory. When information enters the sensory registers it is briefly stored here and then sent to long-term memory or lost. The bottom section (*ventral* portion) of the temporal lobes regulates the recognition of faces and objects (note that this is a different function than recognizing facial expressions). The left portion of the temporal lobe is important for processing auditory information.

■ **Thalamus:** Responsible for the relay of sensory information. Coordinates information with the temporal lobes and serves a primary function in memory.

■ **Wernicke's area:** Located in the rear of the superior temporal gyrus. Believed to be involved in the comprehension of speech.

Before moving on to the next chapter, let's again review the five domains of cognitive functioning.

EXERCISE: COGNITIVE DOMAINS

List the five cognitive domains below:

1. _____

2. _____

3. _____

4. _____

5. _____

Review your answers above. If using an acronym helped you to remember the five domains, you may want to try it again the next time you have to go to the store or need to remember something at work or school.

CHAPTER 3

What Happens to the Brain after an MTBI

Now that we've reviewed some of the basic functions of the brain, we will examine what happens physically to the brain as a result of an MTBI. We will also review the neuropsychological symptoms from the damage and utilize the information presented earlier to match these symptoms to the area of the brain that was damaged.

TYPES OF MTBI

Traumatic brain injury is an acute injury to the central nervous system. Essentially there are two types of head injury: a *closed head injury* and an *open head injury*. In a closed head injury, the skull is not penetrated. The primary damage to the brain is the result of the direct acceleration impact on the skull from an external force. The force causes the brain to move around in the skull, resulting in both *diffuse* (widespread) and *focal* (localized) damage. In an open head injury, the skull is penetrated, resulting in damage to a specific area of the brain. In both types of injury, there is accompanying secondary damage to the brain resulting from swelling, hypoxia (oxygen deprivation), cellular damage, and chemical changes within the cells of the brain.

The consequences of an MTBI are multifaceted and often include altered physiological functions of cells, neurological and psychological impairments, medical difficulties, and other challenges that affect the individual with the MTBI, as well as their family, friends, community, and society in general. An MTBI often goes undiagnosed due in part to the urgent care needed for other, more pressing physical aspects of injury and trauma. The consequences of MTBI can affect an individual across a lifetime and often present new challenges as the individual enters various stages of life.

The literature on brain injuries supports the premise that interventions in mild to moderate cases of traumatic brain injury assist the healing process, resulting in a significant decrease in the number and intensity of symptoms and a more rapid return to work or school. Research is demonstrating that early interventions (including exercises like the ones in this book) may be more beneficial for mild head injuries than for more severe injuries. Unfortunately this is still not a universal belief in the medical community, and these types of interventions are often neglected. As technologies in imaging advance, we are better able to identify the correlation between the symptoms associated with brain injury and the actual parts of the brain that have been damaged. Imaging usually involves the use of either CAT (computerized axial tomography), MRI (magnetic resonance imaging), SPECT (single photon emission computerized tomography), or PET (positron emission tomography).

Direct Contact Force MTBI

Impact or *direct contact injuries* result in specific damage to brain tissue within specific brain regions. Some damage to the brain results from the head directly striking an object, such as a dashboard or windshield. The portion of the brain that hits the object suffers damage. However, this is only part of the overall cause of brain damage from this type of injury. *Acceleration/deceleration injuries* also contribute to this overall injury. This type of injury is most commonly caused by auto accidents. Basically, the head is thrust forward until it comes to a sudden and dramatic stop after striking a stationary object. The brain continues in a forward motion until it strikes the front of the inner skull. This contact of the brain against the front of the skull results in *frontotemporal lesions* (bruising of the frontal and/or temporal lobes). This also causes shearing and tearing of brain tissue and neuron damage as the brain makes contact with rough bony ridges inside of the skull. The resulting brain deficits include difficulty with judgment, inflexibility in thinking, and poor memory, planning, organization, and concentration. Changes in personality and behaviors are also common as all of these skills are controlled by the frontal and temporal lobes. Damage to the *subcortical connections* between the lower area of the brain and the upper hemispheres also results in significant changes in brain function.

Another direct contact force MTBI is the *coup/countercoup injury*. Essentially, this refers to blow/counterblow damage. A moving object connects with the head and briefly dents the skull inward, causing the brain to bounce off the opposite side of the skull. The initial contact area is bruised as well as the area where the brain bounced. Impairment depends on where the blow occurs. Some resulting difficulties include personality changes, perceptual and sensory problems, difficulty with self-expression and balance, and motor difficulties.

Diffuse MTBI

A *diffuse MTBI* results from a mild blow to the head that causes only momentary loss of consciousness and no observable disruption of nerve impulses. This is also known as a *concussion*. However, any time the brain suffers a violent force or movement, the soft, floating brain is slammed against the skull's uneven and rough interior. The internal lower surface of the skull is a rough, bony structure that often damages the fragile tissues within the brain as it moves across the bone surface. The brain may even rotate during this process. This friction stretches and strains the brain's threadlike nerve cells. The cells may even become torn either at the focal point or in other areas in a diffuse injury. Although the stretching and tearing of nerve fibers may seem relatively minor or microscopic, the impact on the brain's neurological circuits is often subtle yet significant.

It is now widely recognized that even a mild injury can result in significant physiological damage and cognitive deficits. This type of nerve damage often heals in time, but there can be long-term repercussions at the cellular level. Nerve impulses often fire at a slower rate and may become less consistent in their functioning. Diffuse damage from an MTBI often results in deficits in attention, slowed information processing, disrupted organization, and impoverished problem solving. Higher-order thinking may also suffer. Self-expression and communication skills may become less consistent, and abstract thinking may be impaired. This diffuse type of brain injury is often accompanied by damage from direct contact force (see figure 3.1 below).

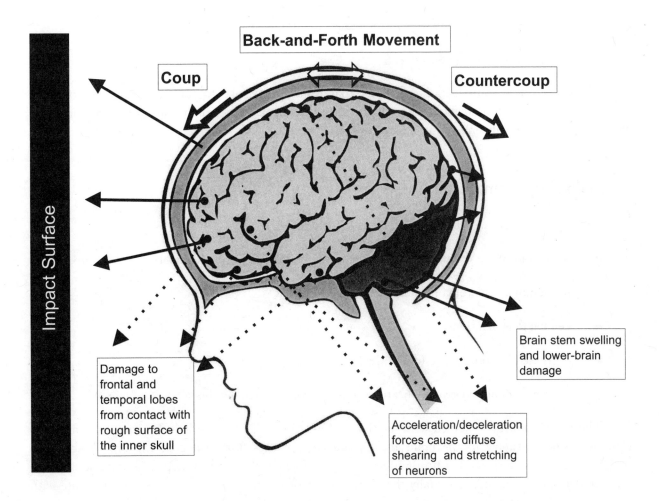

Figure 3.1

THE VARIETIES OF DAMAGE IN MTBI

Outcome and management of MTBI are determined by the severity, nature, and location of the injury. Brain damage may be *primary*, sustained at the time of impact, or *secondary*, the result of subsequent *pathophysiologic processes* (reactions of the body to injury).

Primary Damage

Primary damage to the brain from a traumatic brain injury can take many forms. These include:

- alterations in cerebral blood flow

- diffuse axonal injury (the stretching and tearing of brain tissue, causing short-circuiting throughout the brain)

- intracranial lesions (specific damaged areas of the brain)

- vestibular damage (disruption of the brain's maintenance of the body's equilibrium)

- slowed information processing

There are many consequences of MTBI that result in damage to the brain and temporary or permanent impairment in cognition. Rarely are the consequences limited to one set of symptoms or a disability that affects only one part of a person's life.

Secondary Damage

Secondary factors exacerbating brain damage include:

- neurotransmitter dysfunction (decrease in the brain's release of chemicals)

- intracranial hematoma (localized swelling)

- cellular degeneration

- decreased glucose uptake (diminished brain fuel)

- a variety of pulmonary complications and hypoxia (oxygen deprivation)

The initial injuries combined with multiple secondary insults can result in a variety of symptoms. Diminished blood supply to the brain (*ischemic damage*) causes disturbance in the brain's ability to function. *Axons* (brain fibers that transmit electrical impulses) in the *cerebrum* (cortical or higher areas of the brain) begin to die and eventually the various parts of the brain can no longer communicate with each other. This disconnection is called *diffuse axonal injury*. Diffuse axonal injury is the most common secondary result of an MTBI and manifests itself in subtle ways. Axonal damage can result from damage to a part of the neuronal cell.

The most common cause of diffuse axonal injury is motor vehicle accidents. The acceleration/deceleration force of these accidents results in forceful forward and backward jarring of the head. When the head hits a stationary object, the brain is thrust forward and back in the bony *calvarium* (skull). The inertia of the impact causes the brain to slide and rotate within the skull, resulting in brain *contusion* (bruising) and the rupture of life-giving blood vessels.

HOW MTBI AFFECTS YOUR BRAIN FUNCTION

MTBI can result in a multitude of neurological deficits and usually results in a combination of several. Any cognitive, sensory, motor, or autonomic function may be compromised. These impairments are referred to as *functional,* as they affect the way these processes function. Most of these complications are apparent within the first days or months following injury, depending on the severity of the initial trauma. Some long-term effects might include a variety of cognitive and movement disorders, seizures, headaches, visual deficits, and sleep disorders. Medical complications include, but are not limited to, cardiac and circulatory deficits, pulmonary complications, metabolic changes, nutritional concerns, gastrointestinal complications, musculoskeletal complaints, and dermatologic problems.

The cognitive and emotional consequences of MTBI are equally diffuse. All of these consequences can occur singly or in combinations and are variable in terms of their effects on individuals. Furthermore, they change in severity and *presentation* (how they appear or manifest) over time. In combination, they produce myriad functional problems. Some of the most persistent problems include memory impairment and difficulties in attention and concentration. Deficits in language use and visual perception are common but often go unrecognized or aren't taken seriously. Frontal lobe functions, such as judgment, planning, decision making, problem solving, cognitive flexibility (flexibility in thinking), abstract reasoning, insight, information processing, and organization are often affected to different degrees by an MTBI.

Cognitive deficits are complex in nature and can usually be further broken down and delineated. For example, there are different types of attention (like divided versus alternating attention), various stages of memory that can be affected (like retention versus recall memory deficits), expressive versus receptive language difficulties, and multiple components of complex information processing and sensory perception and processing. These systems are interconnected and thus a breakdown in one often results in a breakdown within the other systems. These deficits can further affect personal and professional social relationships, family dynamics and role functions, and employment and economic independence. These cognitive impairments are further exacerbated by factors such as the severity of injury, the age and general health of the individual, degree and stage of recovery, *premorbid cognitive functioning* (thinking abilities prior to the accident), and a whole array of genetic, psychological, and social considerations. Symptoms of postconcussive syndrome can be further exacerbated by stress (including post-traumatic stress disorder), depression, and anxiety.

Before moving on to chapter 4, which addresses the severity of injury, let's do another exercise.

EXERCISE: MAZE 2

Using a pencil, start in the lower left corner of the maze and find your way to the finish in the upper right corner. Time yourself in seconds and write your time below.

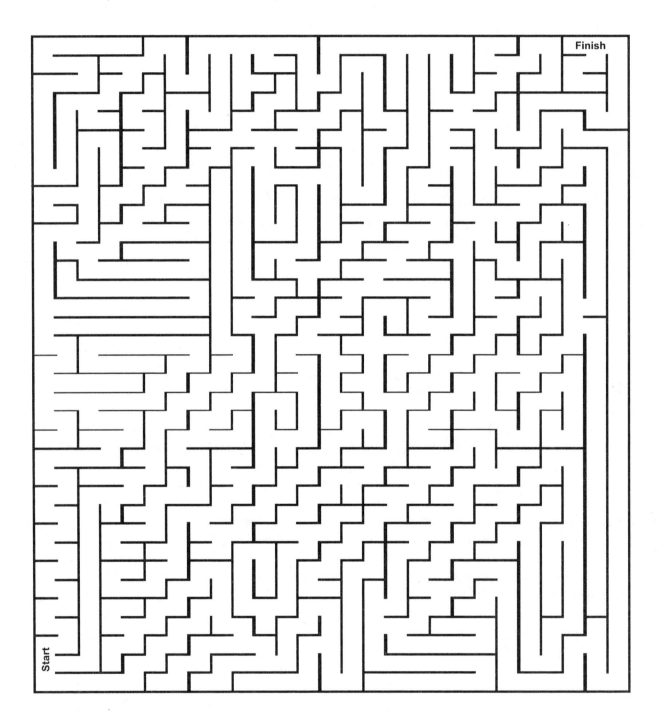

Time: _____ seconds

CHAPTER 4

Measuring the Severity
of the Injury

GAUGING SEVERITY

There are several ways in which the severity of head injuries is measured. These injuries are usually classified by physicians as mild, moderate, or severe. This classification is initially determined by the severity and duration of the coma during the first twenty-four hours after injury and later by the duration of *post-traumatic amnesia* (length of time after the injury before memory function returns).

Glasgow Coma Scale

One method used to examine the level of coma is the Glasgow Coma Scale (Teasdale and Jennett 1974). The Glasgow Coma Scale is a simple scale in which a number of neurological signs and symptoms (motor response, verbal response, eye opening) are measured and then given a rating from 3 to 15 (Jennett and Teasdale 1981). The lower the score, the more cognitive impairment present. A score of 8 or less indicates severe impairment, 9 to 12 means moderate impairment, and a score of 13 to 15 indicates mild impairment (Jennett and Teasdale 1981).

The contents of the scale are as follows:

Verbal Response

- Oriented (5 points)

- Confused speech (4 points)

- Inappropriate or senseless speech (3 points)

- Incomprehensible; makes sounds (2 points)

- None or no speech (1 point)

Motor

- Follows commands (6 points)

- Localizes pain by pulling examiner's hand away (5 points)

- Withdraws from pain by pulling away from the source (4 points)

- Flexion to pain (3 points)

- Extension to pain (2 points)

- No response to pain (1 point)

Eye Opening

- Spontaneous; opens eyes on own (4 points)

- Opens eyes to command (3 points)

- Opens eyes to pain (2 points)

- No eye opening (1 point)

Length of Coma

The duration of the coma also aids in the determination of the *prognosis* (probable outcome). A coma that lasts twenty minutes or less indicates an MTBI. A coma lasting twenty minutes to six hours signifies a moderate TBI. Finally, a coma that lasts over six hours usually indicates a severe brain injury (Lezak 1995).

WHEN IS HOSPITALIZATION NECESSARY?

Even if a head injury is classified as mild, there is still often a need to place the injured person in the hospital for further monitoring and treatment. Hospitalization following an MTBI is usually indicated when there is a Glasgow Coma Score lower than 14. The type and degree of abnormalities found in imaging tests can also determine the need for hospitalization, as can the presence of a skull fracture or the presence of seizures or other unusual neurological symptoms. Hospitalization is also often indicated when there is a significant alteration in mental status, accompanying medical considerations, or suspected drug or alcohol involvement or safety concerns within the home (Horn and Zasler 1992).

Next we will take the information presented earlier about symptom severity and apply it to your injury.

EXERCISE: SYMPTOM SEVERITY RATING SCALE

In order to evaluate the severity of your current symptoms, let's go back to chapter 1. Turn to the section on Symptoms of MTBI where you assigned a number to each of the symptoms listed. Tally the total number of all of the symptoms listed and place the numbers in the space below according to category:

- Emotional symptoms total rating: _____

- Behavioral symptoms total rating: _____

- Physical symptoms total rating: _____

- Cognitive symptoms total rating: _____

- Social symptoms total rating: _____

Now add the five categories above to get a total symptom severity score and place it in the space provided below:

- Symptom severity rating total: _____

Review of the Severity of Your Symptoms

Symptoms resulting from an MTBI can be very specific, influencing only part of your daily functioning. Alternatively, they can be very global and affect a wide range of functions. We have broken down the symptoms of MTBI into five basic categories. This will serve to give you a better understanding of how your MTBI has influenced your life.

In the **emotional category**, your score can range from 0 to 45. If your total score is 25 or above or if any single symptom is a 5, you should seek professional assistance. This can be a doctor, psychologist, or psychiatrist.

In the **behavioral category**, your score can range from 0 to 35. If your total score is 18 or above or if any single symptom is a 5, you should seek professional help. Again, a consultation with a psychologist, psychiatrist, or physician would be the appropriate course of action.

In the **physical category**, your score can range from 0 to 65. If your total score is 38 or above or if any single symptom is a 5, you should seek medical assistance.

In the **cognitive category**, your score can range from 0 to 55. If your total score is 30 or above or if any single symptom is a 5, you should seek assistance from a psychologist, psychiatrist, or physician.

In the **social category**, your score can range from 0 to 25. If your total score is 12 or above or if any single symptom is a 5, you should seek assistance from a psychologist, psychiatrist, or physician.

Now add all of the numbers from each of the five categories. Your score can range from 0 to 225. If your score is 125 or above, you definitely should consult your physician and/or neurologist. If you are scoring in this range, it is probable that you have significant impairment that will require ongoing medical intervention.

EXERCISE: COGNITIVE ANAGRAMS

Before moving on to the next chapter, let's do a quick review of some of the terms that you have learned. Below are words that are scrambled. Unscramble the words to reveal a term related to cognitive rehabilitation. Remember, these exercises are designed to work the areas of your brain that may have been hurt. By working these areas, you will enhance your brain's ability to repair itself.

1. Selves _____

2. BIT _____

3. Scorbutical _____

4. ACT _____

5. RIM _____

6. Brumal _____

7. Snipe _____

8. Nesses _____

9. Daimon _____

10. Renal _____

Check your answers in appendix C.

Now that we have explored the dynamics of traumatic brain injury, we will next look at how to successfully negotiate the medical system and communicate with your health-care providers. Before we move on to chapter 5, let's do another maze exercise.

EXERCISE: MAZE 3

Using a pencil, start in the lower left corner of the maze and find your way to the finish in the upper right corner. Time yourself in seconds and write your time below.

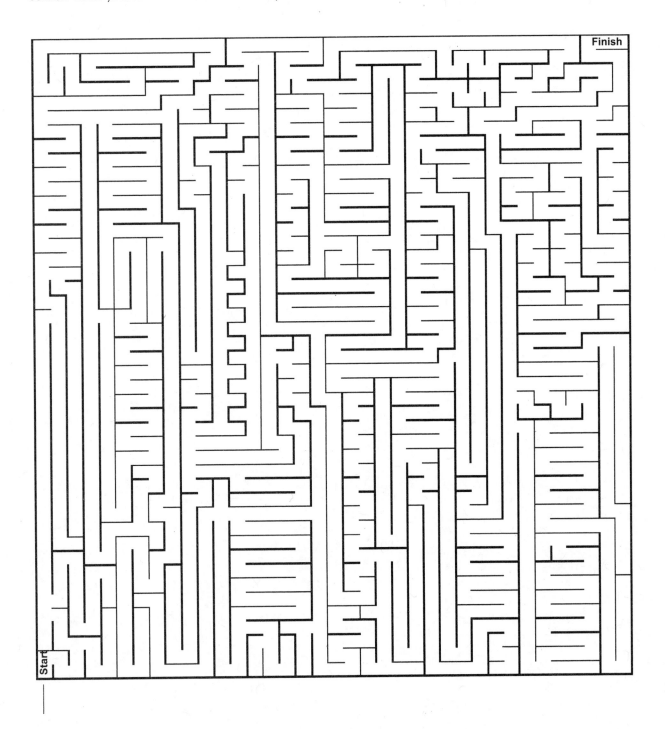

Time: _____ seconds

CHAPTER 5

Setting Goals

Before moving on to the actual rehabilitation portion of this book, it is important that you establish some goals for your recovery. This chapter will teach you how to formulate real and achievable goals based on the symptoms that you recorded as problematic for you in chapter 1. Let's do another maze exercise and then we'll get busy on working up some goals.

EXERCISE: MAZE 4

Using a pencil, start in the lower left corner fo the maze and find your way to the upper right corner. Time yourself in seconds and write your time below.

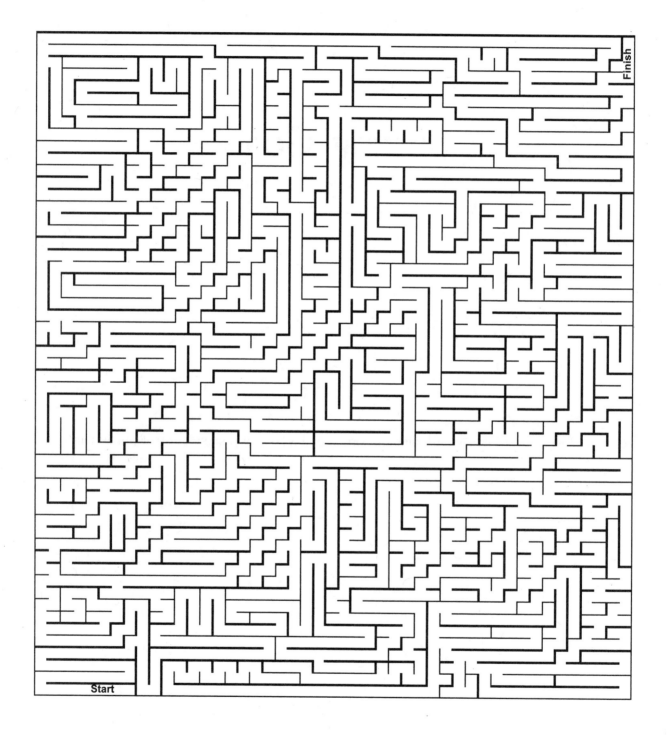

Time: _____ seconds

SET GOALS FOR YOURSELF

One of the most important steps that you can take toward recovery is to create realistic and attainable goals. This chapter will teach you how to do just that.

This will involve a two-step process. You will first focus on the identification of goals using the list of symptoms that you came up with in chapter 1. Next you'll develop very specific, concrete goal statements. Remember, you've already taken a leap forward by making that list of symptoms in chapter 1, ranked in order of severity so you can see how much the symptoms are influencing your life. After reviewing the symptoms, your first step in establishing your goals will be to list them in objective, behavioral terms that will allow you to measure your success. Now let's move on to the exercise itself.

EXERCISE: ESTABLISHING GOALS

Reproduce the symptoms list you created in chapter 1.

1. _____

2. _____

3. _____

4. _____

5. _____

6. _____

7. _____

8. _____

9. _____

10. _____

11. _____

12. _____

13. _____

14. _____

15. _____

16. _____

17. _____

18. _____

19. _____

20. _____

21. _____

22. _____

23. _____

24. _____

25. _____

In this exercise, your task is to convert the above symptoms into realistic goals. Let's start with the example of memory. If you listed memory as a problem area that you were concerned about, then in part I below, you might initially come up with the following goal: "Improve my memory."

Although this is an admirable goal that most people will identify with, it is not stated in a way that will allow you to recognize when the goal has been achieved. In part II you'll work on better ways to state your goals. In the memory example, you might begin by thinking about situations where you feel that your memory can be improved. Do you have more difficulty now with recalling names or do you have trouble in memorizing numbers? How often do you now encounter these problems with your memory and where does it usually happen?

By answering these types of questions and better delineating and defining the problem, you can gain some sense of control over the dilemma, and be in a better position to implement goals and strategies to face the challenges ahead. As an example, the general goal of "improving my memory" can be better defined as "improving my memory when grocery shopping." This is done by answering the question "Where do my memory lapses usually occur?" Perhaps you have become dependent upon a written grocery list and would like to return to the use of a mental list. Your goal can be further delineated to, "My goal is to remember 80 percent of the items that I need at the grocery without bringing my list into the store with me."

You now have a goal related to memory that is well-defined and set up in such a way that it is measurable and you will know when it is achieved. As these types of memory goals are achieved, they can be rewritten and tailored to allow you to accurately gauge your progress. Remember, goals are a process and they will change and grow as rapidly as you do during your recovery from your MTBI.

We will start with the first five symptoms that you listed, as these are the symptoms that are most troublesome for you. Remember to think your goals through and to take them a step at a time, just like a runner who is training to run their first marathon by establishing achievable benchmarks. First they may run two miles and then five. Before they know it, they are up to ten and then fifteen miles. Eventually the goal of the marathon will be met, but only in a realistic, step-by-step, achievable approach.

Before you fill in part I below, look at the top five symptoms on your list. Based on those symptoms, list five goals that you have for your recovery from your accident. In part II, restate your goals in language that is specific and attainable. For example:

Part I: Improve my attention.

Part II: Increase the length of time that I am able to focus on reading a book by one minute each day for five consecutive days.

Part I: Initial Goals. Now it's your turn. Choose these goals based on the top five items on your symptom list.

1. _____

2. _____

3. _____

4. _____

5. _____

Review the goals you listed above. How will you know when you have reached your goals? Under what circumstances and when do the symptoms occur? Where do they occur? Carefully think through the goals above.

Part II: Restated goals. Restate your goals in quantifiable and attainable terms.

1. _____

2. _____

3. _____

4. _____

5. _____

USE YOUR GOALS AS A GUIDE

The goals that you listed above should serve as a basis for working through the rest of this book and making advances in the areas that mean the most to you. If there are certain areas that you feel you are having real difficulties with, you can spend extra time going through those portions of the book.

It may be that you have more than five goals for your recovery. Of course, that is okay. However, I discourage you from overwhelming yourself with a lot of goals. Start off small and build slowly as you go. Though you have only listed five goals here, you can certainly come back later in the book, or even when you have finished the book, and create more goals.

At the end of the book we will come back to these goals for a final assessessment.

Before moving on to chapter 6, let's work the brain a little more.

EXERCISE: NUMBER SEARCH

Find a quiet place that is free of interruptions and time yourself while doing this exercise. Complete the number search below. Number sequences go in all directions, including backward and diagonally. Time yourself and write in the number of minutes that it took you to complete it below. Check your answers in Appendix C when finished.

1	2	7	9	3	5	1	2	1	2	8	0	4	2	7
0	1	4	6	0	2	3	8	7	1	1	9	6	4	9
4	6	6	3	3	2	5	4	3	6	8	1	4	5	7
2	8	1	6	9	3	8	1	4	3	6	0	2	6	4
1	6	0	0	5	8	9	2	6	7	4	3	8	1	6
2	4	7	9	5	3	1	1	0	3	8	4	2	0	6
3	4	7	6	0	4	8	1	4	6	1	1	7	8	3
5	1	5	9	7	4	5	2	7	7	6	3	0	2	7
3	6	8	3	1	2	7	4	4	7	7	2	3	2	1
7	2	4	9	7	3	0	4	3	7	3	9	0	1	5
9	2	4	5	3	2	2	1	6	7	6	4	9	0	2
2	5	9	2	1	1	2	3	8	1	9	1	1	1	9
2	5	8	8	2	5	5	9	2	7	0	9	4	9	3
1	6	4	8	0	9	0	1	1	4	1	9	2	5	8
4	1	7	5	3	9	3	2	3	7	5	9	8	7	2

12793	01647	48146	91857	95528	36901
43681	36831	32086	46109	45610	39528
39147	75910	10908	95123	31974	47629
21637	12952	31286	46823	12327	13589
28169	47148	39550	38191	35379	73901

Time: _____ minutes

CHAPTER 6

Managing Your Medical Care

In this chapter you will be provided with some general suggestions about communicating with your doctor and other members of your medical team. Your physician is the person with whom you will address concerns about diagnosis, treatment, and prognosis. If asking a doctor questions is a source of anxiety for you, you may often leave the doctor's office with unanswered questions. Different people have different relationships with their doctors. Some doctors are willing to form a more collaborative relationship and welcome your input into treatment and medication decisions. Others may become offended if you dare "question" their wisdom. It is important that you choose a physician who fits your preferred style. I recommend that you consider the following information to assist you in getting the most out of your doctor visit.

CHOOSE ONE PRIMARY-CARE PHYSICIAN

The first step in the management of your medical care is to choose one primary-care provider whom all other doctors report through. He or she must be willing to coordinate your overall care and monitor your medications. It's easy to get involved with many health-care providers and to begin to lose track of specific details, such as who prescribed which medication and for what purpose. With a head injury, it can be even more difficult to track orders, medications, appointments, and referrals due to your cognitive impairments. Having a primary doctor can make it easier to negotiate the complexities and frustrations involved in your health care. Your doctor can coordinate referrals and medications and maintain the necessary records, which you are always welcome to obtain. Remember, you are the consumer and can negotiate specific components of your care. Don't hesitate to directly ask your primary-care physician if he or she is willing and able to take on the responsibility of coordinating your overall care. It is essential to your health that your medical treatment be done in an efficient and organized manner.

Prepare for Your Appointments

When you visit your primary-care physician or any other professional, it's a good idea to do some preparation beforehand. It often helps to write down your questions and to bring a list of medications and other health-care providers treating you. This should also include a list of your medical team's addresses and phone numbers. Whenever you see a practitioner for the first time, always obtain a business card and keep these cards organized in a central location. Be prepared to initially answer a large number of questions associated with your health concerns. It's best to reply as succinctly as possible and to take time to formulate an answer before responding. At all your appointments, write down what the provider says so you can refer to it later. Ask about alternative treatment methods in an effort to understand all your options.

If You Don't Know, Ask

Remember, don't be afraid to ask your doctor questions about your health care and medications. You are the one placing the prescribed medication into your body and the one undergoing the evaluation and treatment processes. You therefore have the right to ask your doctor questions and learn as much as you can about the procedures and medications that are prescribed for you. Before making a medical decision, always ask about all your alternatives. This usually involves doing a little research on your own. The Internet can be a rich resource for this. Participating fully in your care and learning what you can from your physician can help you develop a trusting relationship with him or her. You are hiring your physician as an expert consultant for the care of your personal health and to advise you on all aspects of your medications, from the proper use to any side effects you might experience. Your pharmacist is also a good resource, available for consultation regarding your prescription medications.

Have Your Primary-Care Physician Review Your Medications

The initial appointment with any health-care provider should always involve a "brown bag session." This refers to bringing in all of your medications for review. Once you have chosen a primary-care physician that you trust to coordinate all of your care, have that person review your current medications. Make your doctor aware of any medications that you receive from other physicians or that you may be taking over the counter. Also make them aware of any allergies that you might have and what a typical allergic reaction involves. Always ask about any side effects that a new medication may have or any special instructions that you may need to be aware of. If you develop a new symptom after starting a new drug, it's probably a safe assumption that the drug may be causing the symptom. Report this to your doctor. Ask your physician about alternative medications that might be available, and always try to limit the number of medications that you are taking. However, do not adjust your dosage or discontinue any medications on your own. Consult your physician prior to making any changes in your medication.

If a new drug is added, ask if it can replace an existing drug. Gain an understanding of the typical dose of the medication and let your physician know that you would like to start on the lowest dose possible. It is always better to start low and go slow. With injury to your brain, you are more susceptible to the effects of drugs. As we age, metabolism slows down and we usually need less of a medication to do the intended job. Don't take a drug any longer than is necessary. Make sure you have a clear understanding of how the medication is to be taken and the proper dose. Finally, get rid of any old drugs that you're not currently using.

Your pharmacist can also be a good source of information. Take the time to establish a relationship with him or her. Ask questions. Usually an individual will appreciate that you respect their wisdom enough to consult them on an issue. Ask the pharmacist to provide you with any literature that might be available on the medications that you are taking.

Now that we have addressed some of the considerations with your general medical care, we will do another maze. Then we will continue with a discussion of some of the key players involved with your neurocognitive rehabilitation program.

EXERCISE: MAZE 5

Using a pencil, start in the lower left corner of the maze and find your way to the upper right corner. Time yourself in seconds and write your time below.

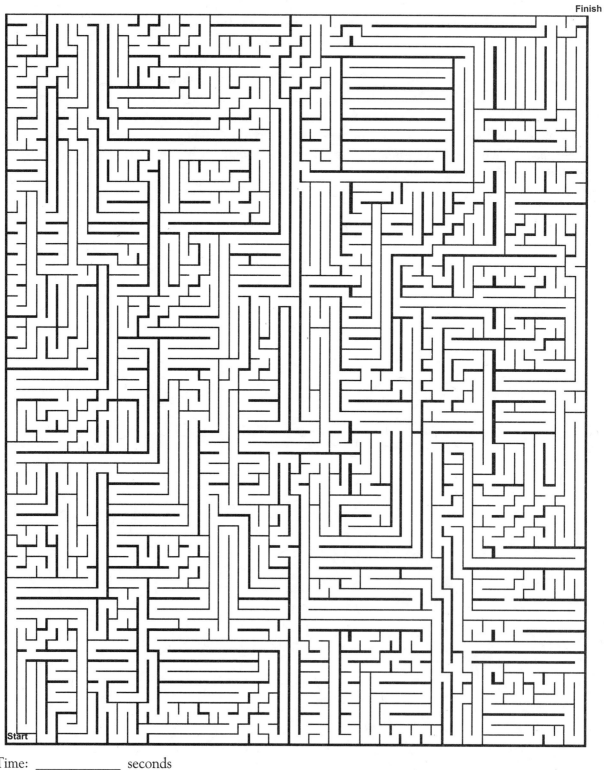

Time: _____ seconds

YOUR NEUROCOGNITIVE REHABILITATION TEAM

Conventional neurocognitive rehabilitation involves many disciplines. Each discipline has a specific background and strategies to offer in the recovery process. Below is a list of some of the more common disciplines. The practitioners you see will be determined by the particulars of your injury.

- **Neurologist:** Neurologists are medical doctors who specialize in conditions of the *central nervous system* (brain and spinal cord). They will often act as coordinators of rehabilitation services. They are an integral part of the diagnostic process, as they are the ones that order imaging and other tests that are essential in your diagnosis. Additionally, your neurologist will prescribe any medication you may require.

- **Neuropsychologist:** Neuropsychologists specialize in measuring brain and behavior relationships through the use of empirically validated instruments. They assist in diagnosing the areas of the brain that have been affected by injury or disease and in offering strategies for treatment.

- **Occupational therapist:** Occupational therapists focus on the functional aspects of neurocognitive remediation. Treatment focuses on safety, driving, social skills, and the management of everyday responsibilities. Their training is similar to that of physical therapists, with a primary focus on the upper body functioning.

- **Physical therapist:** Physical therapists are trained in techniques to decrease pain and increase strength and mobility. They often treat neck, back, and limb pain and other whiplash injuries. Specific techniques include the use of electrodes, ultrasound, ice packs, hot packs, and exercise.

- **Speech and language therapist:** Speech therapists work to resolve communication, swallowing, and hearing impairments. Approaches to neurocommunications include interventions to treat language deficits.

- **Vocational therapists:** The primary focus of vocational therapists is in developing the skills that are necessary for the return to work. Therapy focuses not only on developing the skills necessary to return to work, but also on exploring alternative occupational options. Pet therapy is another technique commonly used by vocational therapists.

THE NEUROLOGICAL EVALUATION

A thorough neurological evaluation should involve a comprehensive history, including a family history of neurological disorders so that genetic influences can be considered. It should also include an examination of current medications, a review of current symptoms, a comprehensive medical workup, and a comprehensive neurological workup. The medical and neurological workup might include:

- Neuropsychological testing

- X-rays

■ Neurological imaging, such as computerized axial tomography scans (CAT), magnetic resonance imaging (MRI), single photon emission computed tomography (SPECT), and positron emission tomography (PET)

■ Electroencephalogram (EEG) to look at the electrical activity of the brain

■ Electromyogram (EMG) to measure activities of muscles

■ Blood workup (some of the more common areas of evaluation include thyroid functioning, vitamin levels such as B_{12}, electrolytes, glucose level, liver function test, and heavy metals screening, to name a few)

■ A lumbar puncture to check for infections within the central nervous system

■ A cranial nerve examination

■ A motor system examination

■ A mental status examination

■ A sensory examination

Diagnostic Techniques

There are many diagnostic methods that may help your physician and other health-care professionals further diagnose and treat your injury. The use of these options will also help to determine the type and seriousness of the injury. The following review is intended to familiarize you with some of the more common techniques used with neurological disorders and injuries.

X-Rays

Skull X-rays are almost always done immediately after the injury to evaluate damage to the skull. The initial detection of fractures of the skull will allow the medical team to focus on the areas of the brain that may be the most damaged or prone to secondary damage. Although X-rays have limited ability to capture the damage to the brain, they can identify areas of intracranial pressure (pressure in the skull) and the presence of foreign bodies within the brain.

CAT or CT (Computerized Axial Tomography)

The level of sophistication in imaging that we currently have began with the CAT or CT in the early 1970s. The technology of the CAT allows the diagnostician to view specific brain regions and the blood supply within the brain in order to distinguish damaged brain areas. In cases of severe injury, a CAT will usually be ordered upon admission and repeated regularly to gauge the progression of recovery and to monitor the development of any secondary injuries.

MRI (Magnetic Resonance Imaging)

The MRI is a technology that was developed within the past two decades. Three-dimensional images of the brain are produced through the use of a strong magnetic field. Images are much more detailed than those found with CAT, making the MRI able to detect more subtle brain insults. The newest technology involving MRI is the functional MRI. This technique allows the mapping of the brain's activity by means of detecting changes in the brain's metabolism and oxygen uptake.

SPECT (Single Photon Emission Computerized Tomography) or PET (Positron Emission Tomography)

SPECT and PET are imaging techniques used to detect cerebral blood flow and brain metabolism. As different areas of the brain are used during the imaging process, the changes in the brain's activity are imaged in a color representation of activity. The use of this technology is limited in that it is expensive and requires the injection of radioactive glucose or radiotracers.

Lumbar Puncture

A lumbar puncture is the method used to obtain cerebral spinal fluid for further study. The fluid is drawn directly from the lower spine with the use of a thin needle. The study of the spinal fluid can assist in the diagnostic procedure by revealing any infections and by measuring the intracranial pressure.

Angiogram

Angiograms are used to detect any abnormalities in the vascular integrity of the CNS. A dye is injected into a blood vessel and X-rays are taken after the injection. This allows the examiner to view the vascular system of the brain in real time and to detect any injury or defects.

Electrophysiological Studies (EEG)

EEG studies provide information on the electrical functioning of the brain. Small electrodes are placed on the scalp and electrical activity is recorded in a graphic format. The procedure is most often used in the differential diagnosis of seizure activity.

Now that you have a grip on what you should expect out of your doctor and what you should get in a full neurological evaluation, we will move on to the physical aspects of MTBI in the next chapter.

CHAPTER 7

Physical Aspects of
Traumatic Brain Injury

The first area of functioning that we will examine is the physical aspects of MTBI. Although most of the physical aspects of brain injury are beyond the scope of this book because they require a comprehensive evaluation from your physician, we will offer a brief overview and suggestions about some of the more common physical challenges after head injury. If I could identify one central recommendation that pertains to all of the physical aspects of MTBI, it would be to seek medical advice about your symptoms. These physical signs are your body's way of telling you that something is wrong, so don't hesitate to consult your physician. Before we move on to the specific physical consequences of MTBI, let's complete our search exercises with a symbol search.

EXERCISE: SYMBOL SEARCH

Complete the symbol search below. Symbol sequences go in all directions, including backward and diagonally. Time yourself and write in the number of minutes that it took you to complete it below. Check your answers in appendix C when finished.

!	@	*	>	#	%	!	@	!	@	<	?	$	@	*
?	!	$	&	?	@	#	<	*	!	!	>	&	$	>
$	&	&	#	#	@	%	$	#	&	<	!	$	%	*
@	<	!	&	>	#	<	!	$	#	&	?	@	&	$
!	&	?	?	%	<	>	@	&	*	$	#	<	!	&
@	$	*	>	%	#	!	!	?	#	<	$	@	?	&
#	$	*	&	?	$	<	!	$	&	!	!	*	<	#
%	!	%	>	*	$	%	@	*	*	&	#	?	@	*
#	&	<	#	!	@	*	$	$	*	*	@	#	@	!
*	@	$	>	*	#	?	$	#	*	#	>	?	!	%
>	@	$	%	#	@	@	!	&	*	&	$	>	?	@
@	%	>	@	!	!	@	#	<	!	>	!	!	!	>
@	%	<	<	@	%	%	>	@	*	?	>	$	>	#
!	&	$	<	?	>	?	!	!	$	!	>	@	%	<
$	!	*	%	#	>	#	@	#	*	%	>	<	*	@

!@*>#	?!&$*	$<!$&	>!<%*	>%%@<	#&>?!
$#&<!	#&<#!	#@?<&	$&!?>	$%&!?	#>%@<
#>!$*	*%>!?	!?>?<	>%!@#	#!>*$	$*&@>
@!&#*	!@>%@	#!@<&	$&<@#	!@#@*	!#%<>
@<!&>	$*!$<	#>%%?	#<!>!	#%#*>	*#>?!

Time: _____ minutes

HEADACHES

One of the most common symptoms experienced after an MTBI is headache. For patients with the least damage, headaches are often the most severe symptom. Headaches can range in both intensity and the type of pain (from mild to severe and from dull to sharp). There are more than a dozen classifications of headaches; however, there are five types that are primarily associated with MTBI. We will review these types of headaches and the associated symptoms. Use this section to identify the type of headache you experience so you can relate this information to your neurologist or primary-care doctor. The five types of headaches most likely to affect you as a result of MTBI are:

- migraine

- post-traumatic

- tension

- cluster

- analgesic rebound

Migraine Headaches

Migraine headaches normally last from four to seventy-two hours. The pain is located at the forehead or temple and is characterized by a throbbing. This throbbing pain may be accompanied by nausea, vomiting, numbness, muscle weakness, and sensitivity to light, sound, or smell. Intensity may increase with activity, and the headache can often be resolved with sleep. Migraines can be triggered by emotional stress, physical activity, the menstrual cycle, irregular sleep, irregular meals, and trigger foods. Some migraines are preceded by an aura consisting of blurred vision, flashing lights, or a brightness. Onset may also be signaled by mood swings, fatigue, and an increase in thirst, food cravings, or energy.

Post-traumatic Headaches

Post-traumatic headaches can occur months or years after an MTBI. These headaches may resemble tension headaches or atypical migraines. They are associated with a burning or tingling sensation and pain that increases in intensity with even a light touch. The rigorous diagnosis criteria for these headaches are too extensive to list in their entirety here. For more information, contact your physician.

Tension Headaches

Tension headaches are typically the result of facial or back pain, often the result of whiplash. Tension headaches associated with MTBI are frequently the result of injury to the vertebrae, ligaments, neck tendons, or jaw. Because they cause intense pressure in your head, they are considered pressure headaches. Typical triggers include worry, stress, overwork, poor posture, and poor ventilation. Onset is normally late in the day, so these headaches may prevent sleep. Degree of pain varies and often these headaches are not debilitating. Tension headaches may be episodic, occurring less than fifteen times per month, or chronic, lasting from fifteen days to six months. Chronic tension headaches are often associated with depression.

Cluster Headaches

Cluster headaches are related to migraine headaches. These headaches are extremely severe and are associated with injury to the back of the neck and nerve damage. Pain is intense and often penetrates behind the eye and affects one side of the face. The headache duration is between fifteen minutes and three hours and the pain may move from one side of the face to the other during the course of the headache. The headache may be triggered by nicotine, alcohol, overwork, or extreme emotion.

Analgesic Rebound Headaches

Analgesic rebound headaches are associated with withdrawal from extended usage of pain relief medications (analgesics). These headaches can be severe and not limited to a specific area of the head. Symptoms include nausea, difficulty concentrating, depressive symptoms, irritability, and restlessness.

Causes and Treatments

Headaches are often the result of other conditions, including whiplash, depression, vertigo (loss of balance), and cognitive difficulties. Headaches after an MTBI cannot necessarily be linked to psychological symptoms prior to the accident. Additionally, there is often symptom overlap with headaches. You may experience multiple headache types simultaneously or may alternate headache types over the course of a week or a month. Your treatment team may include your neurologist, orthopedist, dentist, ophthalmologist, physical therapist, and psychologist. Treatment may include medications or you may opt to try cognitive behavioral therapy, hypnosis, or biofeedback. Always discuss your headaches with your neurologist or primary-care physician.

WEAKNESS

General weakness in the arms or legs is a common result of MTBI. This effect is similar to the effects of a stroke. You may experience *hemiplegia*, which translates to "half paralysis." Essentially, this means that there is damage to one side of the brain. The result of the damage to this one side of the brain is that the opposite side of the body is weakened. For example, if the left side of your brain sustains damage, whether bruising or a blood clot, your right arm and leg will exhibit signs of weakness. In this example, your right arm and right leg will be weak because the left side of your brain has suffered injury.

In cases where damage to the brain is more widespread and deeper in the cranium, *triplegia* may be experienced. Triplegia means that three limbs are affected by the brain damage. The damage will occur in one arm and both legs. Initially, both arms may exhibit signs of weakness; however, after some recovery, one arm will be nearly normal while the other arm and both legs remain weak and spastic.

Typically, the hand is more strongly affected by brain injury than the elbow or shoulder. The hand may continue to be weak and somewhat clumsy after good recovery elsewhere in the body. Your muscles may remain strong, but the joints may not cooperate in moving the muscles. Active reflexes may result in *clonus*, a spastic movement of the muscles. For example, after you make a sudden movement, your hand or foot may continue to move about involuntarily. This spastic movement may cause your joint to slip into an abnormal position. If the joint does not return to a normal position and stiffens, it may affect the future functionality of the muscle.

The weakening of muscles results in stiff arms that are either straight or sharply bent at the elbow joint. The legs are typically straight with the toes pointed. This positioning may result in stiff joints and the rehabilitation team must take great care in preventing or relieving this stiffness so as not to cause further damage. Most likely you will be involved in either physical or occupational therapy to cure the muscle weakness in the arms and legs.

POOR BALANCE

The coordination of movement is controlled by multiple brain systems (see chapter 2). Compared to a stroke, which is normally localized, trauma tends to be more widespread. For that reason, brain injuries usually affect coordination and strength by traumatizing various sections of the brain that normally work together to coordinate movement. Sometimes the impact is restricted to coordination. If you have both weakness and clumsiness, it's difficult to do something as ordinary as rising up from bed. The lack of balance causes your head to fall forward or slip to the side as soon as you rise. Simultaneously, the body slumps. As muscle tone improves, you regain the ability to hold your head up, then sit. Eventually the muscle tone improves in your legs and your trunk, enabling you to first stand and then relearn to walk.

As mentioned, balance is impacted by multiple systems of the brain. One of the primary issues related to balance is limb perception, or *proprioception*. Prior to your injury, you were completely aware of where your body was positioned in relation to the world around you. Now, it may be difficult for you to know how far to reach your arm out to pick up your drink or how far to extend your foot forward when taking a step. This loss of perception has a dramatic effect on balance.

Also, balance is tied to the *vestibular system*. The vestibular system is made up of the balance organs located under the thick part of your skull close to your ear. Included in this area are your hearing organs. These organs are delicate and easily impacted by brain injury. When your vestibular system is injured, sudden movement of your head results in dizziness. The lack of functionality of this system inhibits balance and thus your ability to sit, stand, and walk. You can relate this to a time when you have had an ear infection—the world seems out of balance and your gait uncertain. A similar but less dramatic comparison may be the sensation you experience when changing altitudes or just after landing from a flight or even the sensation you feel after an extended cruise.

A physical therapist will work with you to regain your strength and coordination. As you relearn to walk, you will rely on your therapist for physical support. You'll use a wheeled frame, sticks, and possibly splints for your joints and feet. Your recovery will be dictated by your perseverance and regained muscle strength. This may be a slow process and it will be critical to build your endurance but not strain your muscles. Your physical therapist will be your coach in this portion of your rehabilitation.

SEIZURES

Seizures are characterized by a sudden discharge of electrical impulses and may be isolated to one area of the brain or generalized and diffuse. If seizures occur only after brain injury and are recurrent, the diagnosis is *post-traumatic epilepsy*. Typically, seizures are not associated with mild traumatic brain injury, but rather moderate to severe brain injury. As a result, this discussion of seizures is limited. Seizures are normally associated with damage to the temporal lobes, but they can also occur with damage to the frontal, occipital, or parietal lobes. Seizures are more frequently exhibited in those with a familial disposition to seizures, childhood meningitis, or a history of alcohol or drug abuse. It is absolutely imperative for your neurologist to be involved if you suspect seizures. While seizures cannot be cured, they can be controlled with medication. Additionally, you can limit your exposure to alcohol and caffeine and ensure that you do not become fatigued. You must be compliant with your prescribed medications, and it is imperative that you discuss driving with your neurologist. Again, it is absolutely essential that you work with your neurologist if you suspect any seizure activity.

SEXUALITY

As unromantic as it may sound, sexuality originates in the brain—specifically, the hypothalamus and the brain stem. If you sustain an injury to these areas of the brain, you may find that your sexual desires are repressed or nonexistent. Conversely, you may experience heightened and inappropriate sexuality if you sustain an injury to the frontal lobe. This type of injury is less common than damage to the hypothalamus and is usually associated with moderate to severe brain damage.

Sexual interest may also be impacted indirectly by brain injury. That is to say, a loss of concentration, emotional stressors, fatigue, medications, and so on may cause sexual dysfunction. Nerve impulses may be misinterpreted or not interpreted at all. Touch to the breasts, genitalia, and other erogenous areas may be unbearable due to heightened sensitivity.

This topic may be somewhat uncomfortable for you to discuss with your doctor. However, you can link this particular symptom with other symptoms you may be experiencing (fatigue, stress, lack of concentration) and to medications you are taking. Your doctor may refer you to a psychotherapist, urologist, or gynecologist for further evaluation. It is important to discuss this issue openly with your partner. Eliminating the stress of sexual disinterest and the impact on your partner will help relieve some of your anxiety. You may also want to consider marital therapy to facilitate discussing this issue openly and work on restoring your sexual interest. Together with your partner, you can explore relaxation techniques to use as a couple or create a romantic environment to stimulate sexual arousal.

FATIGUE

Another common symptom or side effect of MTBI is fatigue. Diagnosing the cause of your fatigue is difficult if not impossible since this symptom correlates to so many other symptoms associated with MTBI. In addition, we live in a chronically fatigued society that has become defined by the do-it-all syndrome. Regardless of the cause, fatigue associated with MTBI seems to leave none of the reserve energy that you previously relied upon when you were exhausted. With MTBI, reserve energy is nonexistent.

To compound the fatigue problem, sleep disturbance may be a new problem for you since your injury. When you are overtired, it is often more difficult to fall asleep and to stay asleep. Additionally, pain associated with your injury may awaken you. Other disturbances, like noise, may also disrupt your sleep. You may attempt to overcome your fatigue by using caffeine, which ultimately compounds your sleep woes. In the past, you may have gotten an energy boost from sugar, exercise, or naps, which now only serve to heighten your fatigue.

Fatigue tends to exacerbate the other MTBI symptoms you are experiencing. Your cognitive processes are further slowed by fatigue, and your memory and concentration are also hindered. You will notice decline in efficiency and an increase in irritability when you are fatigued.

Consider the medications you are taking and at what time of day you take each one. Your physician may be able to help you schedule your medication times to minimize sleep disturbance. Or there may be some flexibility in medications so that you can switch to a medication that has less impact on your sleep patterns and tiredness.

You can minimize the effects of fatigue by concentrating on your most intense responsibilities during your most energetic times (typically mornings). It's also very important to learn your limitations and take rests prior to becoming overexhausted. Although it may be hard for you to admit, it takes significantly longer for you to overcome extreme exhaustion than it did prior to your injury. It's critical that you learn to stop and rest before reaching this state. Naps may be useful to keep you energized during the day and may actually improve your night sleep.

There are tricks that can help to work around your fatigue. Don't hesitate to elicit help from your family in managing tasks. Find ways to minimize the complexity of everyday activities. For example, use automated bank systems to pay regular monthly bills. This not only eliminates the risk of forgetting the bill, it also helps ensure the correct amount is paid and gives you one less thing to worry about as you concentrate on healing. There are many strategies that you and your family can enlist to help minimize your fatigue. Eliminating fatigue as much as possible is key to minimizing the other physical symptoms described in this section.

Sleep Time and Quality

In regards to fatigue, one of the most important things to take into consideration is the amount of sleep you are getting and the quality of that sleep. It is important to stick to a schedule for bedtime and waking up. Fatigue will compound the problems you are suffering from. A lack of sleep will compound your fatigue. There have been many volumes written on sleep because it is such a problem for so many people in our modern society. If you are having problems with sleep, I would recommend that you speak with your physician. Undoubtedly there are suggestions he or she can make to help you. However, there are several bits of advice I can give you here to help alleviate your symptoms in the meantime.

For the most part, it is best to avoid sleep medications if at all possible. Studies have shown that your body has a more difficult time entering REM (rapid eye movement) sleep when you take medications. REM sleep is very important, as it is during this stage of sleep that your body enters into a deep restful state. Without enough REM sleep, you are guaranteed to continue feeling tired. Relying on sleep medications can also turn into a habit that is difficult to break. It is far better for you to try to put yourself on a reliable sleep schedule. Speak with your physician about developing this type of routine.

You should also avoid the use of alcohol as a means of getting to sleep. In fact, it is better if you limit your intake of alcohol throughout the process of your recovery. While recent studies have shown that a limited intake of alcohol has certain health benefits, people suffering from an MTBI should really try not to drink too much. Alcohol has a very pronounced effect on your cognitive function and it should be avoided for the most part. In terms of sleep, alcohol does more harm than good. It may be that you feel it is easier to get to sleep after you have had a drink. Unfortunately, your body doesn't rest nearly as deeply when it is busy trying to process the alcohol. If you are going to drink at all, I would recommend drinking several hours before you plan to go to bed.

EXERCISE

With your recent injury, your body's metabolism has probably changed. You may find yourself gaining weight due to decreased activity, or you may require more nutrients and calories to assist your brain in healing. But remember, calories do not necessarily equal nutrition. To help your body heal, eat mostly nutrient-dense, minimally processed foods. Your essential organs, such as your liver and pancreas, may have more difficulty in processing nutrients right now. Exercise is not only a good way to strengthen your body and improve circulation, but it will also assist your body in reestablishing its normal metabolism. It increases your metabolism so that food is processed by the body more quickly, thus absorbing more nutrients. This will greatly enhance your recovery process.

MOVING TOWARD REHABILITATION

This chapter closes the part of the book on the physical aspects of MTBI. It is now time to start your rehabilitation process. The following chapters are built to help you start to regain your cognitive function and cope with the emotional issues that MTBI may have brought up for you. Work well, and good luck.

CHAPTER 8

The Senses

We will start the section on the cognitive aspects of MTBI with an overview of the senses. The senses are the first step in cognition. They serve as our receptors for all the varied stimuli of the outside world. As a result of MTBI, a person will often experience changes in their senses and will sometimes become overly sensitive to sound, light, heat, or cold. These changes can be the result of either alterations in the brain's ability to process sensory information or direct damage to the sensory receptors (such as your eyes or ears). If you are experiencing changes in your senses, it is imperative that you undergo a complete medical evaluation. In this chapter we will examine the senses and how they connect you to other people and the world around you.

THE COMPLEXITY OF THE SENSES

Sensory perceptual functioning is the foundation of all of the other cognitive functions. Because the senses are so fundamental, altered or damaged sensory perception affects a person's ability to perform both complex intellectual tasks and simple skill-oriented responsibilities. Sensory dysfunction slows your brain's ability to think and your ability to interact with the external world. Due to these factors, a malfunction of your senses can magnify other deficits caused by the MTBI. So, it is a good idea to be aware of any sensory dysfunction you may have.

An overview of the senses will begin the process of illustrating the wonderful complexities and intricacies of the brain. The brain is organized in a hierarchical manner where one function serves as the foundation of similar, more complex functions. Your senses are the first step within the process of attention, and attention is the first step in proper memory functioning. The simple process of carrying on a conversation begins with the reception of complex auditory information followed by translation into meaningful words and phrases. Along with the processing of words, we also process the nuances accompanying the words: the cadence of the words, inflection on individual words and syllables, the tone, and the nonverbal gestures. These are all processed within different areas of the brain and later consolidated to form a comprehension of the complete message. Based on this comprehension, we then utilize the motor, memory, attention, and expressive language areas of the brain to respond. All of this occurs in seconds, without a thought given to the actual process.

Given the importance of the sensory perceptual system, we will discuss all of the areas, beginning with hearing.

Hearing

Sound is initially detected by the ears. Sound waves, which are detected by the eardrum, cause small bones within the ear to vibrate. As a result, fluid pressure within the inner ear is altered, causing some 16,000 tiny hairs per ear to react. This activation relays an electrical signal to the brain, where the distribution of those hairs is mapped onto the surface of the brain. This allows you to differentiate among the thousands of sounds you are exposed to on a daily basis. Attention is especially critical with hearing. In any given situation, you are exposed to multiple sounds. For example, picture yourself carrying on a conversation with a friend as you walk through a crowded mall. You are able to engage in that conversation while blocking out the sound of all of the other voices around you. You are able to ignore the sound of people's shoes clicking on the floor, phones ringing, and the music playing in a store nearby. The brain has a wonderful ability to filter out unwanted sounds and focus in on the desired sound. Some have speculated that the inability to filter out sensory stimuli may be the underlying cause of schizophrenia. Just as with vision, there are different parts of the brain designated for different jobs in processing sound. Sounds are located by the brain stem and further processed and identified by the auditory cortex. Complex patterns of sounds (language) are committed to memory. Memory for sounds is located throughout the auditory cortex and other areas. This memory is further tied into emotional memories associated with the sound patterns.

Taste and Smell

Taste is initially detected by the tongue via the taste buds. Just as you perceive only three primary colors, you are able to detect only four primary tastes: salty, sour, bitter, and sweet. Each person has a different number of taste buds on the tongue. The more taste buds, the more sensitive to taste a person is. You may be more or less sensitive than other people. The nose is also involved in taste. *Retronasal olfaction* is the term given to the nose's ability to detect flavors within the mouth. Taste is therefore a combination of nose and tongue. In both taste and smell, what is really happening is that you are detecting hundreds or even thousands of molecules in the air or in liquid. These molecules are converted to electrical impulses that are transported to the olfactory bulb within the brain. A partial or complete loss of smell following an MTBI indicates damage to the *orbitofrontal* area of the brain. The orbitofrontal area is the region of the brain within the forehead. The first cranial nerve (the olfactory nerve) runs along this area of the brain. Damage that is severe enough to damage this nerve will also have repercussions in the orbitofrontal brain region. We will explore the functions of this area of the brain in much more detail, as it is one of the most common areas to become damaged after an MTBI. The good news is that it is also one of the areas of the brain that is the most receptive to rehabilitation with exercises such as mazes and number searches. That's a great reason to do another maze right now.

EXERCISE: MAZE 6

Using a pencil, start in the lower left corner of the maze and find your way to the upper right corner. Time yourself in seconds and write your time below.

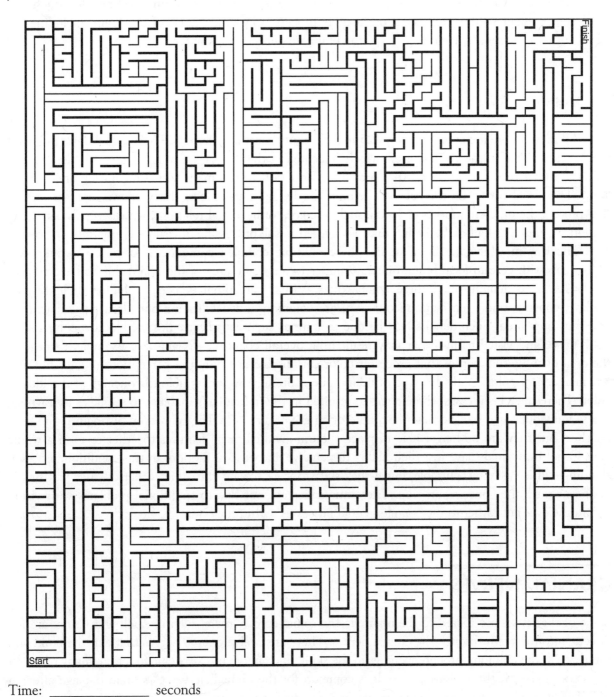

Time: _____ seconds

Touch

Touch is a wonderfully complex sense. The organ that acts as the initial detector of touch is the skin, which is the largest organ of the body. There are at least six types of sensors that detect touch and many types of sensations that make up touch (such as temperature, pain, pressure, and proprioception). Proprioception is the unconscious ability to detect movement and spatial orientation (for example, where the hand is in relation to the mouth when eating). Touch moves from the point of contact on the skin via an electrical impulse up the *dorsal* (back) side of the spinal cord into multiple areas of the brain. Patterns mapped within the brain help us to identify the specific message. In blind people, touch and other senses adapt so that they are more acutely processed by visual areas of the brain, including the visual cortex. The sensory locations within the brain are outlined in chapter 2.

Vision

All in all, there are approximately 125 million photo receptors per eye. These visual detectors relay an electrical signal to the visual cortex, which is located in the rear of the brain. Therefore, the eyes are only the initial receptors of vision that provide information to the many visual-processing areas of the brain. The visual cortex (in the back of the brain) is divided into at least thirty known separate regions that process the different aspects of vision, such as color, form, spatial relations, wholes versus parts, and motion. As much as half of the brain's mass is devoted to the processing of visual information.

The way in which the brain unifies these multiple complex components of vision is unknown. Individuals with certain focal brain injuries (injuries to a specific area of the brain) due to head trauma or strokes have demonstrated these complexities. Visual perceptual defects, including difficulties in reading, copying, and even facial recognition, are common and debilitating but often go undiagnosed and thus untreated. Such deficits may be due to injuries such as *ischemia* (loss of blood supply) to the optic nerve and visual pathways or may result from overall cognitive slowing. For example, damage to the area of the visual cortex that processes color can disable not only the perception of color but also any memory for color. With this type of injury, one is literally no longer able to conceive of the idea of color. There have been cases where a stroke resulted in the individual's inability to see faces as a whole. These individuals can see and describe a nose or an eye or a mouth. They can even distinguish one from another. But they are no longer able to place these individual facial features together to form a whole face. Other individuals have lost their ability to perceive and process motion. In this condition, a person standing still is easily recognizable, but if they start to walk toward the afflicted person they will simply disappear until they once again stop. These anomalies are not due to traditional problems with vision within the eyes but rather to the complex visual processes within the brain.

CRANIAL NERVES

Some of the senses are routed to the brain via the spinal cord. Others, such as smell and vision, are fed directly into the brain through the cranial nerves. There are twelve cranial nerves that exit the brain and run through the cranium through openings in the skull. Each nerve has a specific function, many of which are associated with the various senses. It is common for the cranial nerves to sustain damage after an MTBI. Damage to any of the cranial nerves may be due to potential lesions in a number of locations, including the nerve itself, the cortex, and deep within the brain in areas such as the thalamus and the brain stem.

The cranial nerves are listed below, along with their function.

1. **Olfactory nerve:** Controls smell; runs across the orbitofrontal region of the brain; malfunction often indicates frontal damage

2. **Optic nerve:** Controls vision

3. **Oculomotor nerve:** Controls eye movement and pupil dilation

4. **Trochlear nerve:** Controls eye movement

5. **Trigeminal nerve:** Controls head and facial somatosensory information (touch, temperature, pain, pressure); also controls chewing muscles

6. **Abducens nerve:** Controls eye movement

7. **Facial nerve:** Controls muscles involved in facial expressions and somatic senses from the ear; also involved in taste in the front of the tongue

8. **Vestibulocochlear nerve:** Responsible for balance and important in hearing

9. **Glossopharyngeal nerve:** Controls taste in the back of the tongue and somatosensory information in the mouth and throat areas

10. **Vagus nerve:** Controls motor and sensory information of internal organs and glands; controls autonomic functions such as heart rate and digestion

11. **Spinal accessory nerve:** Controls and coordinates the movement of the head

12. **Hypoglossal nerve:** Controls tongue muscles

EXERCISE: TESTING YOUR CRANIAL NERVES

Now that you know the names and functions of the cranial nerves, let's test them. These tests will help you understand how the cranial nerves work. These tests are not meant to replace an actual clinical examination but will serve to help you to gain a cursory knowledge of nerve functioning and whether you might need a formal examination.

You will need to get a family member or friend to perform the given tasks below. Have them read the directions below and record their observations in the space provided.

1. Olfactory Nerve _____
   Gather several items with distinctive smells (for example, cinnamon, chocolate, and coffee). Have your partner smell each item one nostril at a time. Is one nostril able to detect the odor better than the other? The olfactory nerve is actually a pair of nerves, and it is possible for only one of the two nerves to become damaged. The right nerve controls the right nostril and the left nerve controls the left nostril. It is also possible to have partial damage to both nerves.

2. Optic Nerve _____

Make an eye chart like the one you see at the doctor's office. Include letters of various sizes. Have your partner try to read the lines at various distances away from the chart.

3. Oculomotor Nerve _____

Test the oculomotor and trochlear nerves together with the abducens nerve (see number 6, below).

4. Trochlear Nerve _____

Test the trochlear and oculomotor nerves together with the abducens nerve (see number 6, below).

5. Trigeminal Nerve _____

The trigeminal nerve has both sensory and motor functions. Test the sensory part of the trigeminal nerve by lightly touching various parts of your partner's face with a piece of cotton or a blunt object. To test the motor part of the nerve, tell your partner to close their jaws as if biting down on a piece of gum.

6. Abducens Nerve _____

The abducens, oculomotor, and trochlear nerves control eye movement and pupil dilation. Check the pupillary response (oculomotor nerve). Look at the size of the pupils of your partner's eyes in dim light and also in bright light. Check for differences in the sizes between the right and left pupils.

Hold up a finger in front of your partner. Tell your partner to hold their head still and to follow your finger. Slowly move your finger left to right and then up and down. Your partner should be able to follow the movement of your finger with smooth movements of the eyes. If your partner is having problems with eye movement, it is possible that both the abducens and trochlear nerves are damaged.

7. Facial Nerve _____

The motor part of the facial nerve can be tested by asking your partner to smile and frown. Have them show you their teeth. The sensory part of the facial nerve is responsible for taste on the front part of the tongue. Try a few drops of sweet or salty water on the front of the tongue and see if your partner can taste it.

8. Vestibulocochlear Nerve _____

The vestibulocochlear nerve is responsible for hearing and balance. Stand behind your partner and have them close their eyes. Gently rub your thumb and forefinger together about four inches from the ear. Do this first for one ear and then the other. Have them say left or right.

9. Glossopharyngeal Nerve _____

Test the glossopharyngeal nerve together with the vagus nerve (see number 10, below).

10. Vagus Nerve _____

Determine if your partner is able to taste food and drink normally. Have them eat and drink and observe the swallowing reflex. It may indicate damage to either of these nerves if your partner has problems swallowing.

11. Spinal Accessory Nerve _____
    Test the strength of the muscles used in head movement by placing your hands on the sides of your partner's head. Apply light pressure and have them move their head up and down and from side to side.

12. Hypoglossal Nerve _____
    Have your partner stick out their tongue and move it up and down and from side to side.

If you show deficiencies in any of these areas, you need to see a neurologist for a complete evaluation.

The next chapter will look at attention and the ways that it affects every other part of your cognitive function. You will also be given some exercises and strategies to improve your attention.

CHAPTER 9

Attention

In this chapter we will focus on attention and look at some ways for you to improve in this area. Since your MTBI, you've probably found that it is more difficult for you to focus on simple tasks. Things like reading the newspaper in the morning or understanding simple math problems may seem much more difficult. Attention is the act of focusing on something (especially on some mental activity) so that you can later use the information that you were focusing on. For example, if you make an appointment to get a dental checkup, there are lots of things that you have to pay attention to before you can get to that checkup. You need to remember the time of the appointment, the doctor's name, and the location of her office. If you don't pay attention to these details, it will be very difficult for you to remember the appointment when the time comes.

As you can see, if you are having problems paying attention to things, it will be much more difficult for you to perform your normal daily routine in a manner that is efficient and effective, because you will find it more difficult to remember the things that you have to do on a given day. Memory is really the centerpiece of good cognitive function, and attention is the foundation of memory. Good memory functioning is the direct result of the quality of attention.

Since your MTBI, you have likely noticed that it has become even more difficult to monitor your own thoughts and behaviors—that is to say, it has become difficult for you to pay attention to what is going on inside your mind. This ability to self-monitor is an important factor in your recovery.

For these reasons, I have started this part of the book with a chapter on attention.

Please be aware that we are now in the cognitive portion of the book. For the purposes of retraining your brain, the exercises on attention, memory, and executive functions will overlap. To improve functioning in any of these three domains, the same neurocircuitry must be addressed. Therefore, I will present exercises related to all three domains throughout the section on cognitive rehabilitation. The brain's other functions, such as language and visuospatial processing, are also dependent upon these circuits within the brain, so this focus on these areas will help set the groundwork for the remainder of the book.

REVIEW OF MAZE EXERCISES

Before we go any further in our investigation into attention, let's review your performance on the maze exercises. The maze exercises measure multiple functions, including attention. This review of the mazes will help you figure out if attention is one of the areas that you need to work on. Let's start by writing in your times in the space provided below. Compare your times with that of a control group.

Maze 1 time _____ (located in chapter 2)

- 47 seconds or less = normal or no impairment

- 48–75 seconds = mild impairment

- 76–119 seconds = moderate impairment

- 120 seconds or more = severe impairment

Maze 2 time _____ (located in chapter 3)

- 65 seconds or less = normal or no impairment

- 66–95 seconds = mild impairment

- 96–147 seconds = moderate impairment

- 148 seconds or more = severe impairment

Maze 3 time _____ (located in chapter 4)

- 58 seconds or less = normal or no impairment

- 59–82 seconds = mild impairment

- 83–127 seconds = moderate impairment

- 128 seconds or more = severe impairment

Maze 4 time _____ (located in chapter 5)

- 82 seconds or less = normal or no impairment

- 83–135 seconds = mild impairment

- 136–189 seconds = moderate impairment

- 190 seconds or more = severe impairment

Maze 5 time _____ (located in chapter 6)

- 87 seconds or less = normal or no impairment

- 88–151 seconds = mild impairment

- 152–202 seconds = moderate impairment

- 203 seconds or more = severe impairment

Maze 6 time _____ (located in chapter 8)

- 179 seconds or less = normal or no impairment

- 180–326 seconds = mild impairment

- 327–466 seconds = moderate impairment

- 467 seconds or more = severe impairment

If you have found that attention is an area that you are having some problems with, then you'll need to focus on this chapter more closely. Even if you find that attention is not an area that you are having a lot of difficulty with, I still encourage you to work through the rest of the chapter. You may find some of the information and exercises useful.

TAKE A LOOK

There is one more thing that I would like to have you do before you move on. Have a look at the picture below. There is no need to pay great attention to it at this point, but I will be using it to illustrate a point later in the chapter.

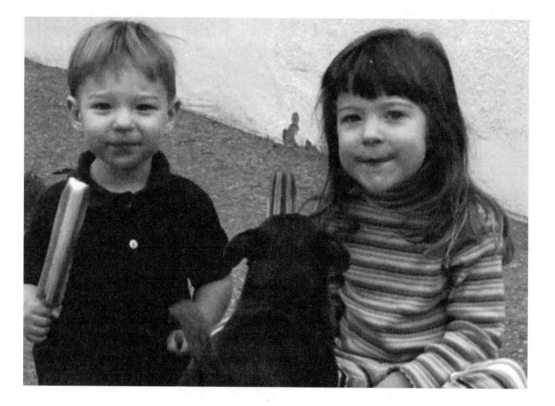

TUNING IN TO ATTENTION

As you now know, attention is an extremely important component of memory and the other cognitive functions. In fact, attentional deficits as the primary cause of memory impairments have been well documented throughout the literature. Attention takes conscious effort. To absorb a piece of information into memory and later be able to recall that information, you must first pay attention to the information. In this portion of the book, you will learn to retrain your attention and to target it in an efficient, effective manner. Prior to your head injury, you probably could pay partial attention to something and later recall it without much effort. Now it may be difficult to rely only on this passive attention to form memories. You may notice that something as simple as paying attention takes more effort, or perhaps you just notice the changes in attention as poor memory recall. Because your brain is healing and reshaping itself, it's necessary to give the information that you want to remember your full attention and to choose the type of attention that you would like to apply.

Given the changes in attention due to a head injury and the importance of attention in memory functioning, it's important to "pay attention to attention" when focusing on something that you wish to remember. There are different types of attention and different levels of intensity that can be applied to your attention.

Types of Attention

There are six different types of attention described by Stankov (1988). Let's have a look at these before we move on.

1. **Concentration (sustained or focused attention):** The application of mental effort in a purposeful, sustained manner (like that used in reading). Concentration is not the same as simple attention because it involves the ability to purposefully direct your attention for a sustained period of time, whereas simple attention usually involves brief periods of focus.

2. **Vigilance:** The ability to detect rarely occurring signals over a prolonged period of time (such as watching for falling stars). Vigilance involves the ability to sustain your attention when there is only occasionally occurring stimuli to pay attention to.

3. **Divided attention:** The ability to perform two different tasks simultaneously. This can occur with similar sensory systems (listening to two people talk at the same time) or with varied sensory systems (driving while reading a map).

4. **Selective attention:** The ability to attend to one stimulus while blocking out another (reading a book while sitting in a crowded waiting room).

5. **Search:** The ability to find a particular stimulus within the context of similar stimuli, like finding a needle in a haystack (letter, number, and symbol searches).

6. **Alternating attention (attention switching):** The ability to switch from one stimulus to another (completing a task while monitoring the time).

Now that we have reviewed the different types of attention, let's do a few exercises that will serve as examples of these different types of attention. You will be asked to do the exercises again later in the chapter after you have been given some strategies to improve your attention. To start with, just go through the exercises in a relaxed state of mind and do them to the best of your ability. It would be best to first photocopy the exercises so that you can easily complete them again later. If you don't have access to a copy machine, make your marks in pencil so that they can be erased when it is time to do the exercises again.

You will notice that there are only three exercises presented, but there are six different types of attention discussed in this chapter. You will actually use three types of attention in every one of the exercises: concentration, vigilance, and search. In fact, you have been using one of these modes of attention throughout the reading of this book. Do you know which one? If you can't come up with the answer immediately, look back over the definitions of the different types of attention. I think the answer will present itself.

EXERCISE: SELECTIVE ATTENTION

In this exercise, you will be asked to focus on completing one task while other stimuli in your environment are competing for your attention. In order to complete the exercise, you will have to be selectively attentive to the task at hand.

To start the exercise, turn on your television and turn the volume up very high. The sound of the TV will be the competitor for your attention.

Now look at the list below. Circle the number 3 each time that it shows up. Time yourself to see how long it takes you to complete the exercise.

1 5 9 8 7 6 3 0 9 6 7 8 3 0 8 7 8 1 0 3 7 6 5 2 9 8 7 3 9 8 2 5 0 3 7 6 5

1 3 3 7 8 5 1 0 8 2 5 3 7 6 5 1 9 0 4 3 2 9 1 7 6 4 8 7 1 5 6 4 1 0 7 3 9

0 7 4 0 9 1 4 6 2 9 7 5 1 3 6 4 4 8 6 9 4 4 9 8 4 5 4 7 3 4 5 7 9 3 1 5 4

5 8 7 4 5 6 3 2 5 5 6 3 8 9 7 4 1 2 8 9 2 4 3 9 5 7 3 2 4 5 7 9 3 5 8 5 2

Write down the amount of time it took you to complete this exercise here: _____ .

You will notice that it is more difficult to complete this simple task when there is other sensory information in your environment competing for your attention. This is the crux of selective attention: choosing which things you wish to concentrate on and being able to ignore the things that are competing for your attention.

EXERCISE: ALTERNATING ATTENTION

Now we will look at alternating attention. Remember that alternating attention is the ability to switch your attention between two or more things at once. I want you to once again circle the number 3 in the following list of numbers. However, this time, every time a 3 is followed by a 5, I want you to switch to circling the number 6. There is another step to this exercise: each time the number 6 is followed by the number 1, I want you to switch back to circling the number 3. This one is a little tricky, so remember to pay close attention. Again, time yourself and see how long it takes you to complete the exercise.

1 5 9 8 7 6 3 0 9 6 7 8 3 5 8 7 8 1 0 3 7 6 5 2 9 8 7 3 9 8 2 5 0 3 7 6 1

1 3 3 7 8 5 1 0 8 2 5 3 7 6 5 1 9 0 4 3 5 9 1 7 6 4 8 7 1 5 6 4 1 0 7 3 9

0 7 4 0 9 1 4 6 2 9 7 5 1 3 6 1 4 8 6 9 4 4 9 8 4 5 4 7 3 4 5 7 9 3 1 5 4

5 8 7 4 5 6 3 2 5 5 6 3 5 9 7 4 1 2 8 9 2 4 3 9 5 7 6 2 4 5 7 9 3 5 8 6 2

Write down the amount of time it took you to complete this exercise here: _____ .

When you have to switch between two or more tasks the way that you did in this exercise, you will find that it takes more attention to do so.

EXERCISE: DIVIDED ATTENTION

This exercise is built to give you some experience with divided attention, which is the ability to perform two tasks simultaneously. This time, I want you to circle every 2 and every W that you come across while simultaneously tapping your foot in measures of three. Tap one, two, three times, and then pause for one second; one, two, three, then pause for a second, all the way through, while circling 2s and Ws. Again, time yourself in performing this task.

2 9 D M 3 L 0 A V 5 M 6 0 D 2 W B 5 0 X 7 B M 3 B 5 2 C G 4 8 F Y 5

2 H V M D 2 E U 7 8 3 0 P L V W D R 3 7 4 9 F J V N W T 2 A Z 0 8 M

8 S 2 D 0 M 3 K 2 F 5 S 9 W 1 Z 8 B 0 M 3 B F 6 7 G 9 0 V 4 S H 2 M 1

3 J V W 8 C 5 A 8 X 9 2 0 4 M 3 2 6 D J W 7 G F H V C 2 4 3 I F 8 Y 3 4 F

Write down the amount of time that it took you to complete this exercise here: _____ .

While in the last exercise you had to switch between two sets of instructions, in this exercise you were asked to do totally separate activities at the same time.

IMPROVING YOUR ATTENTION

Now that you have a better sense of the different types of attention that you may use in your daily life, let's explore some ways to improve your attention overall. There are four basic principles that you can employ in order to improve your attention. These are:

- Active Effort

- Energy Conservation

- Organization

- Preparation

Before I go on with an explanation of each of these principles, I would like to point out that this section is where you can make real advances in your attention. Up to this point you have been given some assessment tools and some explanations about what attention is. Now it is time for you to actually improve your attention and, by doing this, improve your overall cognitive function. What will follow are some guidelines about how to put these principles into play. The more you use these principles responsibly in your daily life, the more your memory and other aspects of your cognitive function will improve. Remember that in some ways, your mind is like a muscle. If you train it responsibly, it will improve. However, you don't want to overdo it. If you find yourself getting fatigued, take a break and come back to this section of the book later. You can think of the four principles of attention as weights. It is your job to use them effectively and responsibly in order to improve your cognitive muscles.

Active Effort

Before we get going with this section, let's do an exercise that will ultimately help you understand what is meant by active effort.

EXERCISE: ACTIVE ATTENTION VS. PASSIVE ATTENTION, PART ONE

Remember the picture earlier in the chapter? Before you go back and look at it, simply write down what you remember about the picture.

_____

_____

_____

_____

Did you experience some difficulty describing the picture? What within it stuck in your memory by chance? You may notice that you weren't able to recall much about the picture. If this is true, don't worry—you're not alone. Most people can't remember a great deal about a picture when they haven't looked at it for a little while.

Now go back and reexamine the picture. Take time and study it with a new mind set and with a focus on your attention. Take the time to strategically place your attention on the different details in the picture. Really get into it. Is there a story that the picture is telling? Is there an emotion that it expresses? Look for fine points that you initially didn't notice and then come back here and continue reading.

Have you ever noticed that the more closely you analyze something, the easier it is to remember the details about that thing? It doesn't matter much what it is. It could be a piece of poetry you read, a song you listen to, or the directions to a friend's house. The more effort you put into really trying to absorb the details of any of these things, the more likely you are to recall them later. It has been shown in studies that the more effort people put into remembering a particular set of stimuli when they first encounter it, the more likely they are to remember those stimuli. When a person first encounters any stimuli, their sensory functions start encoding that information in the brain. If a person is consciously putting effort into this process, the neural connections in the brain that store this information will be more sophisticated. That is to say, if you pay attention to the stimuli, you will encode the information better. Put another way, if you pay close attention, you will be able to remember more easily.

On the other hand, you may happen upon a piece of poetry, read over it, and not pay much attention to it. Or a friend might rattle off the directions to her house at a party after asking you to stop by sometime next week. In neither of these cases would you be likely to remember the details of the information you were presented with.

This is the essential difference between *active attention* and *passive attention*. In active attention, you put effort into remembering the details of a given set of information. In passive attention, you simply happen upon information without actually putting much effort into processing it. If you are actively attentive, you will remember more, and if you are passively attentive, you will remember less.

This is not to say that passive attention is bad. In fact, it is an absolutely necessary function of the brain. There are lots of times when it is important that we get certain information in a situation, but it is not required that we commit these things to memory. For example, it is a good thing to notice the price of gas at a gas station, so that you know how much you are spending when buying your fuel. However, it wouldn't do you much good to remember this exact figure for days and weeks at a time. In this instance, you are using passive attention.

In order to understand active attention more completely, let's go ahead and complete the exercise above.

EXERCISE: ACTIVE ATTENTION VS. PASSIVE ATTENTION, PART TWO

In the space below, write down what you remember from the picture now that you have spent some time studying it.

_____

_____

_____

_____

_____

Do you notice a difference? You probably notice that you are able to remember a great deal more detail this time around.

This exercise was designed to give you a hands-on experience as to what it means to employ active attention. If you want to improve your attention, the first step is to put some effort into paying attention. Take this skill with you to your daily life. If there is a meeting at work that you need to remember, really pay attention when the boss announces the time for the meeting. Or, maybe you just want to remember the lyrics to your favorite song better. Next time you hear it, really listen to the lyrics. You will find that this type of daily practice will go a long way toward helping you remember things.

Remember: practice, practice, practice. You can practice being actively attentive at any time. Experiment with it. While driving or walking a familiar route, take the time to notice something that you haven't noticed before. Even if the route is short, there will be an endless array of things that you haven't noticed before. Why haven't you noticed these things before? It's because you did not choose to focus your attention on them. Learn to focus your attention and remember more.

Energy Conservation

Although effort is important in improving attention, minimizing the amount of effort required to complete any given task is also essential. Remember, with brain injury comes fatigue. If you learn to manage the fatigue, your cognition will improve. Effort takes energy. You simply can't go around focusing intensely on everything in your environment; you'll just run out of steam. Remember that you only have so much energy to give. Managing this energy is critical to improving your attention and your memory.

The first step in this is to limit the distractions around you. Distractions take up valuable cognitive energy—energy that you could expend more fruitfully in other places. In any given situation, limit the distractions and concentrate on the task that is at hand. For example, let's say your boss has asked you to do some filing at work. It is not a terribly difficult task, but it is important that you focus on it so that it is done correctly. As you start the filing, you notice that you are becoming tired, and it is getting harder to keep your focus. Then you notice that you have the radio tuned to a talk radio program that is droning on and on. You also notice that you have had to take breaks in order to answer your phone several times throughout the task. You can hear another employee chatting with a friend in the lunchroom.

If you were in this situation, what would you do? What do you think might help you relieve your fatigue and restore your concentration so that you can get the filing job completed? That's right—eliminate those distractions. Turn your radio off. Maybe you can even put your phone on "do not disturb" temporarily until the job is finished. You might even consider asking your fellow employees if they can keep the conversation down or take it outside. Whatever it takes, reduce the distractions in your environment. You will find that this way you will get less fatigued and you will be able to keep that active attention going for a longer period.

The second part of conserving energy is rest. As I have said throughout this book, it is important to rest when you feel that you are too tired to focus your attention on the task at hand. MTBI is going to make your mind tire more quickly. Take frequent breaks in order to help remedy this.

In the example above, another good idea would be to take a ten-minute break before going on with the filing. You might step out and go for a walk or just sit and have a cup of tea. Better yet, try to find a nice quiet spot where you can simply sit and rest. In this way, you are taking a break and eliminating your distractions at the same time. This is bound to go a long way in conserving the fuel for your attention.

Organization

Do you ever feel like you have more to remember and think about than you can handle? After sustaining an MTBI, you may feel overwhelmed with all of the things you have to remember just to get through the day. One way that you can help keep yourself from getting overwhelemed and feeling confused is to get organized.

There are a lot of details that we have to remember every day just to get by in our busy society. You probably have meetings at work and dates with friends, and perhaps you have to take the kids to soccer practice or meet your partner for a drink on Friday night. To remember these things takes attention.

If you are constantly preoccupied with trying to remember the appointments and responsibilities you have to take care of, it will inhibit you from putting your attention toward other things. There is only so much attention that you have to give, so you need to use those limited resources wisely.

Rather than spending your cognitive energy trying to remember what you have to do throughout your day, use some assistive devices to get yourself organized. You may want to buy a calendar and write down all of your appointments in it. You can use your computer or a PDA (personal digital assistant) or just make notes to yourself about what you have to do throughout the day. If you have a cell phone, it may have a personal organization system built into it. Some people even call themselves and leave messages on their own answering machines. Find a method to organize your activities that works for you. I would recommend even writing down the things that you have to do every day or every week. For example, if you have a weekly Tuesday meeting, don't simply take it for granted that you will remember it just because it happens every week. Write it down. That way you are assured to remember the meeting without having to worry about it.

By getting yourself organized and using some system that will help you remember what you have to do, you will be saving your attention for other things.

Preparation

If you are about to engage in a task that you know will take some attention, preparing yourself for that task will help you focus your attention much better when you are actually performing the task. You've heard the saying "be prepared." That is exactly what you need to do in order to use your attention to its fullest capacity.

There are actually two different steps to proper preparation: the *preparatory set* and the *preparatory review*.

Preparatory Sets

There are a number of steps that go into completing any task. For example, the exercises earlier in this chapter asked you to do a number of different things in order to complete them. A preparatory set is basically a list of the steps that go into any activity. Preparatory sets are useful for two reasons. The first is that they give you the chance to break down an activity into its component parts. By doing this, you can more easily focus on the details in the project. The second is that they give you the opportunity to visualize the event before it happens. By doing this, you will find that it is easier to focus your attention on what you need to do when the time comes. Visualizing an event before it happens is a great way to improve your performance in that event.

To create a preparatory set, there are a number of things that you need to do. First you need to break down an activity into its component parts. Think about all of the little things that you will need to do in order to complete your task. Then go through and carefully consider and visualize what it will take to complete each of these tasks.

Let's look at an example to give you a better idea of how to complete a preparatory set.

Tina invited a couple of her friends to dinner. She knew that to make the dinner a success she would have to give it her full attention. Since her MTBI, Tina had been having some problems keeping her attention focused. She decided to prepare for the dinner in order to keep herself on track. She started by making a preparatory set. First she decided what she was going to serve for dinner. Then she started making a list of all the ingredients and all of the steps that went into preparing the food. She laid out the pots, pans, and utensils that she was going to use to make the meal. She began carefully imagining each step and what it would take to complete each part of the meal. Once she felt fully prepared, she started cooking the dinner, using the same steps that she had just visualized.

As you can see from the example above, a preparatory set can be quite simple or quite complex, depending on the task at hand. You can make a preparatory set for any activity that you are about to engage in; it doesn't have to be something as complicated as cooking dinner for guests. For example, look back at the exercises earlier in the chapter. There are several steps to each exercise. One way to improve your performance on these exercises is to first create a preparatory set. Think about each step in the exercise. Don't be afraid to read over the instructions a few times. Once you have a firm grip on what the exercise is asking you to do, take a moment to visualize and rehearse the activity in your mind. Only when you are completely ready should you go forward with completing the exercise.

When you are creating preparatory sets, be as detailed as you can. Make sure that you understand each step in the process before you go on with your activity. You can even write down the steps if that helps you remember what you have to do. In the example above, Tina might have wanted to write down the recipe she was going to use or write down the steps necessary to make the meal. Another thing you may want to do is physically prepare the things that you need to do the work. Remember when Tina took out her utensils, pots, and pans? This is a perfect example of how you might get the things that you need prepared in advance.

The real key is to do whatever you need to in order to focus yourself on the task at hand and make yourself more comfortable with the activity. Thinking about what goes into an activity beforehand can take you a long way toward improving your attention.

Preparatory Review

A preparatory review is a chance for you to look at the activity that you just completed and think about how well it went and how you might improve upon it. In one way, a preparatory review sounds like an oxymoron. How is a review preparing you for the event? This is a bit of a misnomer. What a preparatory review really allows you to do is prepare for the *next* time you do the activity. It is a really useful tool in that it gives you the chance to praise and criticize yourself so that you can perform better next time. Let's see what Tina came up with when she did her preparatory review.

Tina's dinner was a success. Her use of the preparatory set method really helped her focus her attention and make a delicious dinner for her friends. She was proud of her work. However, Tina realized that there were a few things that she could have done better. If she had put in the vegetables a little bit later, they would have come out a little crunchier. If she had taken out the meat a tiny bit sooner, it would have been a little more tender. Overall she was very happy with her work, but it was useful for her to think about the ways in which she could improve the dinner so that she could do a better job next time.

If you do a preparatory review, you are bound to think of a couple of ways that you might have been able to improve upon what you did. In this way, you will know what you have to pay attention to next time to do that much better.

Remember that the preparatory review is not a time for you to tear yourself down. Don't be too hard on what you may not have done so well. Try to be objective and look at what you did clearly, but don't be too harsh on yourself. There is always room for improvement. This is just a way for you to see where that improvement can be made.

REVIEW THE ATTENTION EXERCISES

Now that you have learned about the different kinds of attention and the strategies you can use to improve your attention, I would like to ask you to go back and complete the three attention exercises in this chapter again. Before you start, think about the type of attention that you will be using in the exercise. Also, remember to use the attention strategies in this chapter. Make an effort to be actively attentive during the exercise. Think about whether or not you are too tired to do the exercise now. If so, come back to it later today or tomorrow. Also, remember to eliminate the distractions that will keep you from focusing your attention on the exercise. Are you thinking about what time you have to pick up the kids from piano lessons? Get a notepad and write the time down and put the note in a place where you are sure to see it. That way you can give all of your mental energy to the task at hand. Finally, remember to create a preparatory set before you start, and do a preparatory review once you are finished so that you have a better sense of what you need to do and what you can improve. Record your new scores below.

Selective attention score: _____

Alternating attention score: _____

Divided attention score: _____

Did you notice any change when you applied attention in these new ways? It is very likely that you did. But if not, don't get discouraged. You can improve and you will improve if you just keep practicing. Remember, you can keep working on your attention until it improves.

TAKING IT TO THE OUTSIDE WORLD

Rebuilding your attention is going to take time; there is no way around that. Please don't get discouraged if you do not see immediate progress after doing this chapter. Just keep working on your attention. Take the skills that are in this chapter with you in your everyday life. The more you apply these principles, the more likely it is that your attention will improve.

As I have said throughout this chapter, attention is the foundation of memory. In the next chapter, we will be looking at memory. Remember to take your attention skills with you through the rest of the book so that you get all you can out of it.

CHAPTER 10

Memory

An MTBI almost always results in some kind of memory impairment. In the last chapter, we explored attention and the way that it affects the encoding processes in memory, and we covered several types of retrieval. In this chapter, we will be exploring memory in much greater detail. Encoding is only one part of your memory system. There are several other components of memory and, in fact, there are many different types of memory. In this chapter, we will review how memory functions so that we can identify where in the process of memory you may be experiencing difficulties.

It is now known that the mind is capable of continued growth and retraining. The brain can be exercised and the workings of the mind expanded. Scientists are discovering that the brain is much more adaptable and pliable than once thought. You may have learned, growing up, that people are born with a fixed amount of brain cells and that brain cells do not reproduce. This has turned out not to be the case. In fact, the brain is not only capable of reproducing brain cells, but it can also repair neural networks and rewire neural connections when needed. However, in order for this to happen, a person has to work on it. You have to put effort into the repair of your mind in order to see results. This holds true not only for attention, as suggested in the last chapter, but also for memory and all of your other cognitive functioning. That being said, let's get to work on repairing your memory.

AN OVERVIEW OF MEMORY

Memory is a process by which information is taken in through your senses and then processed by many different systems in your brain and stored for later use (Parente and Stapleton 1993). It is the way your mind keeps a record of your experiences. The value of memory is that you can then call on this stored information for use later and in other parts of your life. Without memory, the coherent experience of your life would be stripped from you.

In some ways, memory is like a vast and complicated filing system in which certain pieces of data are stored in certain places in your mind. It differs from the filing cabinet in your office in that there is no single place in your brain that keeps all of the information that you need to use. Rather, it is like a building full of offices, each of which has one or more filing cabinets. You have access to a great deal of this information if you can learn how to properly store and recall the data.

There is a particular process by which your mind takes raw data (things that you experience in the world) and turns this data into memory. Interestingly, this process happens in three distinct stages. There are also many different types of memory that your mind employs as a means of storing and retrieving this information. It is important for you to have a basic understanding of these different components of your cognitive function so that you can more effectively repair the memory systems that have been damaged by your MTBI.

The Process of Memory

The process by which you actually remember things is fascinating and relatively complex. Most of the time we never even think about this process; it is so natural that we take it for granted. However, since your MTBI, you very likely have been encountering some problems with your memory. Perhaps you have found that it is hard for you to commit simple things to memory, even for a short time. Or maybe you have noticed that you are having difficulty recalling things that you have known all your life and that before your injury were almost second nature. For these reasons, it is important that you now become conscious of the way your memory works. The better you understand the basic underpinnings of your memory function, the more effective you will be at improving your memory.

Memory actually happens in three stages. These are encoding, storage, and retrieval. Let's look at each of these stages individually before we explore the way that they all connect to form memories.

Encoding

Encoding is the process by which your brain develops a "code" to store information once you are exposed to it. It is at this point in your memory function that your brain starts to create neural connections and networks that will eventually become memories. You may remember that in the last chapter we discussed the concept that the more carefully you pay attention to a set of information, the more likely you are to remember it. That is because the better the information is initially encoded in your brain, and the more systems involved in this encoding, the stronger the initial neural networks will be and thus the easier it will be for you to recall the information later. This concept was developed by Atkinson and Shiffrin (1968) and stands today as one of the many models of memory that neurologists still use.

In this chapter, we will be exploring encoding further. As you might imagine, there are many different ways that you can encode information. Likely you will have strengths in some of these areas and weaknesses in others (everybody does). Later on we will be exploring these strengths and weaknesses, and you will learn to use them to your benefit.

Storage

Once information has been encoded in the brain, it immediately starts to be stored. *Storage* is your ability to effectively accumulate memory.

When information is first stored, it goes into your *short-term memory*, or what is often referred to as your *working memory* by neurologists. This is a storage facility for all of the information that you are using right now. For example, if you had to call a department store to see what their hours are, you would first go to the phone book and look up that number. This phone number would then go into your working memory until you walked to the phone and dialed the number. It is unlikely that you would have any need to remember the number after the call, and therefore this information would simply be disposed of.

If you did have a reason to remember the number (perhaps it is your favorite store and you know you will want to call back later for more information), this working memory might be transferred to your *long-term memory*. Long-term memory is all of the information that is stored in your brain for later use. One of the most important ways to transfer a short-term memory to a long-term memory is to rehearse the information that you want to remember. In the example above, if you wanted to remember the phone number, you would likely repeat the number to yourself again and again until you were sure you "had it." This process is called *rehearsal*. There will be more on rehearsal later in the chapter.

Retrieval

Retrieval is the final stage of the memory cycle. This is your ability to recall information. This is the part of the memory process where you actually "remember." There are ways that you can improve your retrieval, but if you are having a problem recalling information, it is most likely that the information was not encoded or stored very well in the first place. It is generally accepted, as I have stated throughout this portion of the book, that the more effort you put into encoding and storing information, the easier it will be for you to retrieve that information. For this reason, we will not be spending a great deal of time on retrieval per se. However, it is important for you to understand and consider retrieval throughout your recovery process. If you are having problems recalling information, it is a sure sign that there is some problem in the earlier stages of your memory function.

Putting It Together

Now let's put all of these stages together. In order to do this, I will give you an example of the way that a memory is built from its first inception to its final recall.

Jim had a lunch date with a friend from work. They decided to meet at a restaurant, but Jim had never been there before. He decided to look online for directions to the restaurant. Once he had located a map and directions, he started to read the directions and look over the map very carefully. At this point, he was starting to encode the information in his brain. He decided that he would pay careful attention to the details of the map and directions so that he could encode the information more effectively.

As Jim was looking over the information, it started to get stored in his short-term memory. However, he wasn't going to meet his friend for several days, so he decided that he had better try to commit the directions to long-term memory. He read the information over and over, rehearsing the directions in his mind. In fact, he even visualized each of the streets he would have to travel down and all of the turns he would have to make. Soon he was quite confident that he had stored this information in his long-term memory.

The day came for the date, and he was quite satisfied on the drive to the restaurant that he was able to successfully recall all of the information that he had stored in his brain earlier in the week. He didn't miss a turn, and the trip to the restaurant was quite smooth.

Types of Memory

As I have said, there are many types of memory. The type of memory you use, and therefore the location where it is stored, depends upon the type of information you are presented with. It is important that you have a basic understanding of the different types of memory. If you are conscious of the type of memory you are using when you first encounter information, the memory will be encoded in your brain much more effectively.

There are three types of memory that I would like you to consider through the rest of this book. While there are many different types of memory, an examination of these three types will give you the base you need to start to improve this part of your cognitive function. The three types are semantic memory, episodic memory, and procedural memory.

Semantic Memory

Semantic memory involves data related to who, what, and why. When you see an old friend in the street, it is this part of your memory functioning that allows you to know who they are and why they are close to you. It is also this part of your memory that allows you to remember bits of poetry, song lyrics, and paintings.

Semantic memory consists of two major subdivisions: *verbal memory* and *visual memory*. We will be discussing these in more detail later in the chapter.

Your semantic memory is the place where you can have the greatest direct impact on your ability to remember. For this reason, most of this chapter will focus on assessing where your strengths and weaknesses are in your semantic memory and will provide exercises for you to improve on or compensate for these weaknesses.

Episodic Memory

Episodic memory acts as the memory for when and where and is controlled largely through the frontal lobes. When you meet an old friend on the street, you might remember the first time you ever met her. This information is coming from your episodic memory.

Some memories are what we call *state-dependent memories*. That is to say, you are more likely to remember a set of information if you are in the same state as you were when the memory was encoded. There are those annoying times when you walk into another room in your house only to forget what you went in there for. Often, if you walk back into the room in which you first had the thought, it will pop back into your mind. This is a state-dependent memory. You have to be in the same state (in this case the same room) as you were when the memory was encoded in order to be able to retrieve the memory effectively. State-dependent memory is a kind of episodic memory.

Procedural Memory

Procedural memory stores information on how to do something. All of the skills that we have learned are recorded in our procedural memory. In essence, our procedural memory is our life's work. These skills may be vastly complicated (like building a computer from scratch) or they may be fairly simple (like riding a bike).

While you can effectively work on any of these parts of your memory through applied conscious effort, the memory type that you are most likely to have a great impact on is your semantic memory, as I mentioned above. Let's have a look at the different components of your semantic memory and how you can start to improve this part of your memory functioning.

THE LEFT BRAIN OR THE RIGHT BRAIN?

Your brain can be divided into two separate hemispheres, the left brain and the right brain. As you may know, each hemisphere specializes in dealing with certain types of information. That is, different types of memory are stored in each of these two parts of your brain.

In 90 percent of people, the right brain is responsible for storing visual information and the left brain is in charge of storing verbal information. You may have heard the phrase, "She is a right-brained person." This has to do with where a person's particular talents lie. In this example, the person would have a great deal of talent dealing with visual information.

As mentioned above, your semantic memory essentially consists of two different subtypes of memory. These are your visual memory and your verbal memory. Your visual memory is your ability to effectively process visual information. If you are really good at remembering directions by looking at a map, then it is likely that you have a strong visual memory. Your verbal memory, on the other hand, is your ability to process verbal information into your memory. So if you are good at reading directions and remembering them, but you are not particularly good with maps, then it is likely that you have a strong verbal memory.

I have already explained that certain types of information are recorded in either the left half or the right half of the brain. It then stands to reason that if you have had an injury to the left side of your brain, it is likely that you are having some trouble with your verbal memory. Or, if your injury was on the right side of your brain, you probably have some problems with your visual memory.

It is important to know where your strengths and weaknesses with visual and verbal memory lie so that you can maximize your strengths and minimize your weaknesses. Take the following quiz to help you determine whether you have a stronger verbal or visual memory.

EXERCISE: VISUAL OR VERBAL MEMORY ORIENTATION

Circle the answer that best applies to you.

1. When I am driving in an unfamiliar place, I:

    a. Follow street signs

    b. Navigate using landmarks or other visual representations

2. When I meet someone new, I:

    a. Focus on what the person is saying (for instance, their name)

    b. Focus on some physical feature

3. In my spare time, I would rather:

    a. Listen to music

    b. Watch television

4. When writing down directions, I prefer to:

    a. Write out verbal directions

    b. Draw a map to follow

5. If I am doodling on a piece of paper, I tend to:

    a. Write words

    b. Draw pictures

6. If I had a choice, I would rather:

    a. Write a poem

    b. Paint a picture

7. If I were going to take a college course for fun, I would rather take:

    a. Review of English Literature

    b. General Photography

8. When watching a movie, I:

    a. Pay more attention to what is being said

    b. Focus more on what is happening

9. I enjoy reading:

    a. True

    b. False

10. In my spare time, I would prefer to:

   a. Do a crossword puzzle

   b. Do a jigsaw puzzle

Tally up all of the times that you circled "a" and all of the times you circled "b" below.

a = _____

b = _____

If the number of "a" responses is greater than the number of "b" responses, then you are probably more verbally oriented. If the number of "b" responses is greater than the number of "a" responses, then you are probably more visually oriented. If the totals are within one point of each other, then you are equally strong verbally and visually.

Once you get a grip on where your memory strengths and weaknesses are, you can start to use this information to your advantage. In many, many cases you can choose the type of memory that you would like to use in order to store information. For example, directions can be given to you visually (through a map) or verbally (via written or spoken instructions). If you play to your strengths and choose the type of memory that you are stronger in, you will be far more likely to remember things effectively.

Let's take this a step further by reviewing the letter, number, and symbol searches that you did earlier in the book.

Review of the Letter, Number, and Symbol Searches

Go back to each of the searches (in chapters 1, 5, and 7) and write the time it took you to complete the exercises in the space provided below.

Letter Search time: _____

Number Search time: _____

Symbol Search time: _____

If you review the answers in appendix C for the three search exercises, you will notice that the answers for all of the exercises were in exactly the same positions. Each puzzle also contained the same number of characters. In this sense, you basically completed the same exercise three different times. The only difference was that the characters changed, and the side of your brain that you were using to complete the exercises changed as well.

Symbols and numbers are both processed by the right side of the brain. As you know from what you've read so far, letters are processed by the left side of the brain. The symbol, number, and letter exercises were designed to help you use the different hemispheres of your brain based on the type of information you were asked to search for. Use the information below in conjunction with the Visual or Verbal Memory Orientation quiz above to make some further conclusions about where your strengths and weaknesses lie.

If you are over the age of fifty-six, you can add two minutes to each of the cutoff times. The results are as follows:

Letter Search:

- 39 minutes or less = normal or no impairment

- 40–53 minutes = mild impairment

- 54–67 minutes = moderate impairment

- 68 minutes or over = severe impairment

Number Search:

- 35 minutes or less = normal or no impairment

- 36–47 minutes = mild impairment

- 48–62 minutes = moderate impairment

- 63 minutes or over = severe impairment

Symbol Search:

- 45 minutes or less = normal or no impairment

- 46–59 minutes = mild impairment

- 60–76 minutes = moderate impairment

- 77 minutes or over = severe impairment

This scale should give you a pretty clear idea as to how impaired your right or left brain may be. If you are having particular problems completing the symbol search, for example, but you did very well on the letter search, then you can bet that you are having problems with your right brain. This also suggests that you will likely have some trouble with your visual memory. If the opposite is true and you did quite well on the symbol and number searches, but did poorly on the letter search, then it is likely that your verbal memory is impaired.

The conclusions that you make here will prove very useful to you as we proceed though this chapter.

Translating Visual and Verbal Memory

In order to improve your memory function overall and improve your quality of life, one of the most important skills you can learn is how to translate visual and verbal memory. What I mean by "translating" is your ability to take a set of visual information and turn it into verbal data, or vice versa. Now that you are aware that you have strengths in certain areas of your memory function, you can start to take advantage of this knowledge. If you are a strong verbal learner, you can start to break visual information down into verbal data. If you are a visual learner, you can develop ways to make verbal information into visual data. Throughout the chapter I have used the example of driving directions as a way to describe the relationship between these two types of memory. You can apply this relationship to many types of information. Almost anything that is said verbally can be depicted pictorially, and the opposite is true as well.

For example, Gustavo worked for a publishing company. He had been asked to make a report of sales for the books in the current season's catalog at the next meeting of directors. He went into the sales database and started to look up the information that he needed to generate this report. He had decided that he would commit the sales figures to memory so that he could present them more effectively. The problem was that all of the data that were available on the sales of the books were in the form of pie charts and Gustavo did not have a particularly good visual memory. So, he decided that he would take this visual information and convert it into verbal data. He started by making a list of all the books and all of the total sales figures for the books. He then made a brief description for each title of where they were sold and by whom. This process made it a lot easier for Gustavo to grasp the information at hand. After a bit of rehearsal, he was able to commit the sales figures and associated information to memory successfully, which allowed for an excellent presentation.

Leticia was a marine biology student who was taking a class on marine life in shallow coastal regions. It was finals week and she was getting prepared for her test. Her teacher had given her a long list of animals and plants to memorize and Leticia was having a hard time with the list. After all, she had a good visual memory and this list was a long way from helping her remember what she needed to know for the exam. Leticia learned through a friend that the local aquarium was having an exhibit on coastal regions. Leticia decided to take her list and go visit the aquarium. By doing this she was able to actually see the marine life on the teacher's list. With this picture in her mind, she was much more capable when the time for the exam came, so she did very well.

With a little bit of creativity, you can do the very same things that Gustavo and Leticia did. Now that you are aware that you can change verbal information to visual information and vice versa, you can start putting this into practice in your daily life. For verbal memory tools, focus on being succinct and to the point. When creating a visual representation, do your best to make it clear and clean. Here is a list of a few things to keep in mind as you translate visual and verbal information:

- **Be creative.** There is almost always a way to translate information. You just have to figure out how to do it. Don't be afraid to be as creative as you want. The goal is to work your memory. Do whatever you need to do in order to achieve this goal.

- **It doesn't have to be complex.** There is no need to make things more complicated than they need to be. The above examples about Gustavo and Leticia include pretty sophisticated ways to translate visual and verbal information. In a lot of cases, simple exercises will work. A list of grocery store items or a sketch of the route to a friend's house can go a long way toward helping you remember.

- **Ask for help.** There are resources all around you for help. Friends, family, and even coworkers are likely willing to help you. You never know, they may get something out of this process as well.

BUILDING MEMORY MUSCLE

Up to this point in the chapter, we have been exploring the different types of memory and the ways that you can take advantage of these different memory types. Now it is time to start actually building your memory muscles. In this part of the chapter, I will give you exercises and strategies that will help you strengthen your memory. These exercises will focus on two areas in the process of memory described earlier: encoding and retrieval. I will start with the memory exercises that are involved in encoding and then move on to those involved in retrieval. However, before doing this, I would like you to read the following passage and commit the items in the list to memory. We will refer to this later in the chapter.

EXERCISE: CLEANING THE ATTIC

Imagine that on a lazy Saturday afternoon, you decide to go up into the attic and do some spring cleaning. In the process of cleaning, you decide to throw away the items on the list below. Take about five minutes and memorize the items that you are going to throw away.

1. Some lamps

2. An old radio

3. A stack of newspapers

4. Some hubcaps

5. An unusable barbecue grill

6. Some old phone books

7. A power drill

8. A hammer

9. An old television set

10. A checkers game

Encoding Strategies

As you already know, the most important place that you can make a difference in your memory is in the encoding process. By this point we have discussed encoding quite a bit, so you should have a pretty firm grip on what it is. If you have forgotten, look over "The Process of Memory" section in this chapter.

The next few memory-building techniques listed will help you further improve your encoding process.

Rehearsal

The most natural way to build your memory muscle is to do repetitions. You may have noticed that when you need to remember a phone number, you will say it to yourself over and over again. This process, called rehearsal, is one of the most important ways that you can encode information more deeply into your memory. It is also one of the essential ways to make a working memory into a long-term memory. Rehearsal is simply the act of doing something again and again until you remember it.

Almost everyone knows what verbal rehearsal is simply because it is such a natural process. However, we may not really recognize other types of rehearsal. Learning to ride a bike is essentially a matter of rehearsal; you do the activity over and over again until you remember how to do it. You may be able to remember a particular type of wine simply by the smell. This is also because you have rehearsed this smell (you have smelled the wine again and again) until it becomes a part of your long-term memory. You can rehearse almost anything.

Since your MTBI, you may have a problem remembering any number of things. Perhaps you just got a new job and you are frustrated because you are having trouble remembering your way around the office. Take the time to rehearse it. Simply walk around the office a few times, taking notice of where the different desks are, who sits at them, and what they do. Use the attention skills that you learned in chapter 9 to make this encoding process even more profound. Maybe you are having a hard time remembering how to get to your best friend's house. Make sure you are using the type of memory (visual or verbal) that suits you best and then rehearse the directions until you are sure you remember them. There is really no end to the difference rehearsing information can make to your memory.

Elaboration

Another way to encode information more deeply into your memory is to use *elaboration*. Elaboration is the process by which you take a set of information and make it as rich and as detailed as you can possibly make it. As you know, different types of information are stored in different areas in the brain. By involving as many of your senses as you can in a memory, you are storing information on that memory in many different areas of your brain. This is immensely helpful for later recall. Because you have involved different areas of the brain, the information is not only ingrained more deeply in your memory, it is stored in several areas of the brain, making it that much more likely that you will later be able to recall the information.

Let's say that you have a list of errands that you need to do and you are afraid you will forget to do them all. You need to gas up the car, do the grocery shopping, pick up your kids from school, and deliver some papers to your accountant. One way to remember this long list more effectively is to elaborate on each of the scenarios. Think of the sound and the smell of the gasoline as it goes into the gas tank. Picture the aisles in the grocery store and the feel of the apples as you pick up each one to test them. Think of how happy you will be when you see the kids, and how relieved you will be when you drop off those papers. Getting all of your senses involved in a memory will really help you to recall it later. What's more, thinking of the emotions that will be involved in the memories can help you to keep them in your mind as well. There is actually a difference between factual memory and emotional memory. Getting your emotions involved will help you store the information in yet another place in your mind.

Imagery is also incredibly important to elaboration. By visualizing the things that you want to remember, you will enhance the encoding of your memory that much more.

Association

Association is the means by which you anchor a piece of information that you want to remember to an existing memory. This may sound a little strange, but you probably already do it all the time. For example, you are having dinner at a wonderful restaurant for the first time and one of your favorite songs comes on the radio. You are thoroughly enjoying the food and the song. Two weeks later, when you are cleaning the floors in your kitchen, it is unlikely that you would randomly recall the dinner. However, if that song came on the radio while you were cleaning, it is likely that you would be reminded of the restaurant and the meal. You might even remember the very taste of the food and the conversation that you were having over dinner. This is because the memory of that occasion has become associated with the song.

You can consciously use association as a means of improving your memory. Perhaps your friend has just introduced you to his wife, and you would like to remember her name the next time you see her. One way to do this is to relate her name not only to her face, but also to your friend's name and face. It is likely that he is so ingrained in your memory that you won't forget him. By associating his wife with him in this way, you make it more likely that you will remember her as well.

Retrieval Strategies

Retrieval is the stage in your memory where you are most likely to actually feel deficits. When you are trying to recall information and you can't, you are likely to feel frustrated. It may be that this is a source of anxiety for you. You may be wondering why it is that your mind isn't working correctly and why it is that you can't store information. In fact, you can store information, it's just that your means to access this information have been temporarily altered. The best way for you to understand this is to grasp the difference between *recognition* and *free recall*. Recognition is your ability to recognize a set of information that you've already been exposed to. Free recall is your ability to actually call this information into your working memory whenever you wish to. In most cases, people who have suffered from an MTBI have no problem with recognition. That is to say, the information was actually successfully encoded and stored in their minds to begin with, but they simply have a difficult time accessing that information at will. It is very likely that this is the case for you. On the other hand, if you actually have problems recognizing items that you have seen before, it is likely that you are not encoding memory correctly to begin with. In order to understand this better, take some time to complete the next step in the Cleaning the Attic exercise that you started a few pages back.

EXERCISE: CLEANING THE ATTIC— FREE RECALL VS. RECOGNTION

Part One: Free Recall

List the items from the attic cleaning exercise presented earlier in the chapter, without looking back at it.

1. _____

2. _____

3. _____

4. _____

5. _____

6. _____

7. _____

8. _____

9. _____

10. _____

Part Two: Recognition

In the list of items below, circle yes or no according to whether each item presented was in the list of ten items that were to be thrown away after cleaning the attic.

1. Some lamps		Yes / No
2. An old stereo		Yes / No
3. A stack of newspapers		Yes / No
4. Navy discharge certificate		Yes / No
5. Some hubcaps		Yes / No
6. A beautiful pink satin jumpsuit		Yes / No
7. An unusable barbecue grill		Yes / No
8. A power drill		Yes / No
9. An old computer		Yes / No
10. A saw		Yes / No
11. An old radio		Yes / No
12. A can of sardines		Yes / No
13. A checkers game		Yes / No
14. A worn-out set of auto tires		Yes / No
15. A chess game		Yes / No

16. A large seashell   Yes / No

17. Some old phone books   Yes / No

18. A pile of eight-track tapes   Yes / No

19. A hammer   Yes / No

20. An old television set   Yes / No

For part one, check your answers against the original list presented earlier. Convert the number you got correct into a percentage by dividing the number of correct answers by ten (the total number of items) and then multiplying that number by 100. So, if you got five correct, you would divide that by ten then multiply it my 100 to arrive at 50 percent. You therefore would have remembered 50 percent of the information that was presented to you. Put the percentage that you obtained in the space below.

Number correct _____ /10 x 100= _____ %

For part two, score the number of correct responses by comparing your performance to the answers in appendix C. Convert the number into a percentage by dividing the number of correct answers by twenty and then multiplying my 100.

Number correct _____ /20 x 100= _____ %

You should have scored significantly higher on the recognition test than on the free recall test. It is likely that you had a very low score on the free recall test—40 to 50 percent—while you may have scored as high as 80 to 90 percent on the recognition test.

This is the typical pattern with people who have suffered from an MTBI. Rest assured, you can encode information, you just have some problems accessing it. If, however, you are having problems with the recognition exercise, I would recommend that you get a thorough memory examination from a neurologist.

Your problems with recall should be temporary. The simple remedy, as I've described in this chapter, is to enhance your encoding. Because you should have no problems encoding, this is an area that you can really capitalize on. The more good information that goes in, the less effort it will take to call on that information when you need to.

However, there are a few strategies that are effective for helping out in the retrieval process. Let's explore these a bit.

State-Dependent Memory

State-dependent memory (Goodwin et al. 1969) is a memory that is contingent upon the state that you were in when the memory was first encoded. This can be either a physical state (a room that you were in when the information was encoded) or an emotional state (being happy when you first encoded the data). Have you ever had the experience of getting up to go do something in another room in your house, and by the time you get to that room, the reason that you went in there has vanished from your mind? This is a state-dependent memory.

In order to use state-dependent memories to your advantage, try to recreate the state you were in when the memory was first encoded. Often, in the above example, simply returning to the room where the thought formed will bring it back to mind. If you were particularly happy when you formed a memory, try to recreate that happiness. In many cases, recreating the state that you were in when you first encoded the information will help your retrieval process.

Associative Recall

As you now know, memory is stored by many different themes in many different places in the brain. Sometimes when you are having a hard time remembering something, you can use things that are associated with that item as a means of jump-starting your memory. Try thinking about things that are associated with the information you want to remember. Do you remember what time it was when the memory was encoded? Are there sensory experiences (sight, sound, taste, touch, smell) that go along with the memory? Sometimes even the category of an object or the properties that are associated with it can spark the memory. Try to be creative and think of all the potential associated information when you are trying to recall something.

Talking to Remember

This is a kind of verbal extension of using associative recall. When you can't remember a thing, it often helps to talk about the things that you do remember about it. For example, let's say you have forgotten the word "apple." (I know this is a simple one, but let's run with it.) In order to bring the word to mind you might say aloud, "A crunchy red fruit that is often used in pies. Lots are grown in Washington." You get the idea. Talk about all of the associated things that go along with the thing that you want to remember.

EXERCISE: TALKING TO REMEMBER

Try practicing your associative recall skills by describing the list of items below. Pretend that you are talking to a friend and you are having a hard time remembering the words, so you have decided to talk them out to help you remember.

- Orange

- Corvette

- Your wedding

- Trip to Bermuda

- High school prom

- Childhood friend

Remember that there are no right or wrong answers here. This is just an exercise to give you an idea of how you might use some associated details to bring the things you want to remember more clearly into focus.

A WORD ON RELAXATION

Before we conclude, I would like to make a brief mention of the importance of relaxation in memory. You may find that you become very tense when you try to remember things but can't. This may be particularly pronounced when you are trying to communicate and can't seem to find the words or when you are having a hard time remembering information that you have known all your life. Please be aware that tension is an enemy of good memory. When you are tense, your mind is wrapped up in a very complex set of physiological responses that inhibit normal cognitive function.

If you want to improve your memory, relax. There are many relaxation strategies in chapter 14. I suggest you employ these when you are getting too anxious to remember clearly.

ADDITIONAL HELP

This chapter should give you a much better grip on the overall way that your memory functions, and the exercises should help you improve your memory. Of course, memory is vastly more complex than what has been described here, and there are many volumes written on it. If you are interested in further improving your memory, I recommend picking up a copy of *The Memory Workbook,* published by New Harbinger Publications. It is a much fuller exploration of the workings of memory and how you can improve it.

As with the rest of the information in this book, the real test is the difference that it makes in your daily life. Remember to take these exercises with you in your daily life. I am willing to bet that if you employ these strategies, you will see a vast improvement in your memory. In the next chapter, we will be exploring your cognitive communication skills.

CHAPTER 11

Cognitive Communication

A primary area of functioning that is often affected by MTBI is communication, which is multifaceted.

According to the American Speech-Language-Hearing Association (ASHA), communication includes listening, speaking, gesturing, reading, and writing in all domains of language (2004a). Therefore you may see your problems with language crop up in any number of areas in your life. It may be that you are having a difficult time communicating your needs to the people in your life. Or it may be that you sometimes have a hard time understanding passages of text that, before your MTBI, seemed very simple to read. As you can imagine, a vast array of communication problems can develop because of an MTBI. The more severe types of communication disruption are beyond the scope of this book and require professional assistance. However, if you have made it this far in the book, you are certainly prepared for the exercises and information in this chapter. This chapter is designed to help you understand how language is an intimate part of cognition and to exercise the parts of your cognitive-communication function that have been impaired by your injury. Some of the exercises are quite difficult, so please be patient and try not to get frustrated. Having said that, let's get started.

LANGUAGE AND COGNITION

According to ASHA, language is "a complex and dynamic system of conventional symbols that is used in various modes for thought and communication" (1983, 44). Based on this definition, we can see that our ability to use language effectively is intimately tied to our ability to think. In fact, language and cognition are interdependent. There are two different ways that problems in this language/cognition matrix can occur. You may have cognitive difficulties that are affecting your ability to process language, or you may have problems understanding language that are leading to a problem in your cognitive functioning. These types of problems are commonly known as *cognitive-communication disorders*. Regardless of the type of problem you are having, exercising the parts of your brain that process language will help you recover.

Let's start by looking at a few of the common changes in cognition that interfere with language:

- Problems with disorganization, inflexibility, and impulsivity

- Impaired attention, perception, or memory

- Changes in the processing of information (rate, amount, and complexity)

- Difficulty processing abstract information

- Difficulty learning new information, rules, and procedures

- Inefficient retrieval of old or stored information

- Ineffective problem solving and judgment

- Inappropriate or unconventional social behavior

- Impaired executive functions

- Disorganized discourse (spoken and written) and difficulty comprehending extended text (auditory and reading comprehension), likely associated with generally impaired organizational functioning

- Difficulty learning new words or other forms of language

If your MTBI has had an impact on your cognitive function in any of these ways (and it likely has), then it is probable that you also have some language impairments that you will have to face as well. It is especially likely that you will face problems with some of the higher-order language processes. Let's do an exercise that will give you an overview of how well your cognitive-communication systems are processing.

EXERCISE: VERBAL ASSOCIATION

Below are a number of items. Write in what the item listed is a part of or associated with.
Examples:

a. Hand is part of the   arm

b. Toe is part of the   foot

c. Nose is part of the   face

Answer the questions in the space provided. There may be more than one answer to the questions.

1. Ballpoint is part of a _____

2. Steering wheel is part of a _____

3. Pedal is part of a _____

4. Foot is part of the _____

5. Knob is part of a _____

6. Page is part of a _____

7. Bulb is part of a _____

8. Limb is part of a _____

9. Speaker is part of a _____

10. Collar is part of a _____

11. Blade is part of a _____

12. Leaf is part of a _____

13. Tile is part of a _____

14. Lace is part of a _____

15. A pip is part of a _____

16. A filament is part of a _____

17. Decimal is part of a _____

18. An oar is part of a _____

19. Iris is part of an _____

20. Cuticle is part of the _____

21. Incus (anvil) is part of the _____

22. Hippocampus is part of the _____

23. Heel is part of the _____

24. Bark is part of a _____

25. A wick is part of a _____

26. Aileron is part of an _____

27. Cones and rods are parts of an _____

28. An inning is part of a _____

29. A stirrup is part of a _____

30. A ripcord is part of a _____

31. A bride is part of a _____

32. Type is part of a _____

33. A pimento is part of an _____

34. A bayonet is part of a _____

35. An inauguration is part of a _____

36. RAM is part of a _____

37. A piston is part of an _____

38. A mouse is part of a _____

39. A cavity is part of a _____

40. A margin is part of a _____

41. A talon is part of a _____

42. A lash is part of an _____

43. A pillar is part of a _____

44. A shingle is part of a _____

45. A treble clef is part of _____

46. A scalpel is part of a _____

47. Corolla is part of a _____

48. A cob is part of an _____

49. A noun is part of a _____

50. A radiator is part of a _____

Check your answers in appendix C. Tally your correct answers. Add six points to your total score, as there are several correct answers to many of the questions.

Total _____

40–50 = above average

30–39 = average

20–29 = below average

0–19 = impaired

Please keep in mind that this test is simply an overview of how your cognitive-communication skills are functioning. It does not take into account different specific areas of language that you might be having problems with. However, the types of verbal associations given in the exercise are indicative of skills your brain would have a problem with if you have experienced any of the cognitive changes mentioned above. If you had problems with this test, then you can be certain that this is an area that you need to work on. Even if you did well on the test, we recommend that you work your way through the rest of this chapter. It is chock-full of information on the way that language is processed in the brain, and it will certainly assist in your recovery.

RECOVERING YOUR LANGUAGE ABILITIES

Unlike some of the other areas of cognitive function addressed in this book, your ability to recover your skills in the cognitive-communication domain is contingent on whether or not you practice these skills. In other chapters, you have been given tools to compensate for problems that you may be having in certain areas by using strengths in related fields. To make a strong recovery in your skills with language, you need to be exposed to language and use it. And you need to do this in several different ways.

Even the simplest language tasks depend on a complex interaction of many different areas in the brain. When language is processed, a vast neural network comes into play that would make even the world's fastest computer look like a horse-drawn carriage being driven down one of today's freeways. Due to this fact, it is almost impossible to isolate the precise areas of your brain that have been damaged in your accident and work on these. However, there are ways that you can work on recovering the damaged part of your mind. As was stated earlier, most of this simply revolves around using your language centers in a variety of different ways. To that end, simply reading and doing the exercises in this book will have helped you to improve your cognitive-communication skills.

Now let's work on some exercises that will further your progress.

EXERCISE: WORD PUZZLES

Below are several verbal puzzles. On each line provided decipher the phrase represented by each brainteaser.

Answer: A stitch in time

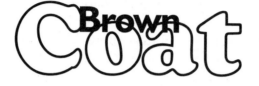

Answer: _____

Coat
Brown

Answer: _____

ATTE(N)TION

Answer: _____

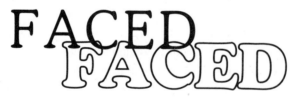

Answer: _____

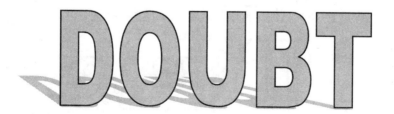

Answer: _____

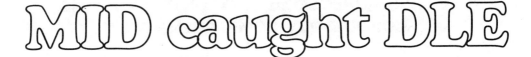

Answer: _____

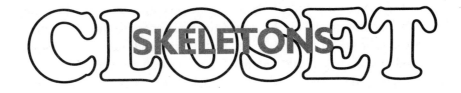

Answer: _____

Check your answers in appendix C.

The answer to each of these brainteasers is a standard American idiom—something that you have heard a thousand times. Although the phrases themselves are common, deciphering puzzles like these is still good training for your abstract verbal reasoning skills. Abstract verbal reasoning is a set of higher-level language skills that allows you to take abstract information and translate it into words. Your higher-level language functions are the ones that were most likely affected by your MTBI. Thus, simply completing exercises like these gives your cognitive-communication skills a bit of a workout.

The Neuroanatomy of Cognitive Communication

We have already discussed the functions of the different parts of your brain. In the following section, we would like to take the time to go into the specific neuroanatomy of your cognitive-communication function. We are going to do this in the form of an exercise. The language in this exercise will be complex. By presenting this information in this fashion, we are actually serving two purposes. The first and most obvious is to simply teach you a little bit more about how your mind works. More importantly, by completing this exercise, you will be working on the very parts of your cognitive-communication function that have been damaged due to your MTBI. The very fact that the material is difficult to understand makes you work your mind a little bit harder to grasp it. We call this process *compulsory comprehension*. By forcing the areas of your brain that are utilized to comprehend this material to work, you will actually speed your healing process. In other words, if information is forced through the broken networks of your brain, your brain will be forced to do something with that information. The process of forcing your brain to route this information will empower your brain to strengthen existing networks and generate new ones.

Having said that, we would like you to take your time with the exercise and try not to get frustrated. For the purposes of recovery, it is not necessary at this stage that you understand every part of this text, but rather that you make a conscious effort to try to understand it.

EXERCISE: PURPOSEFUL PRONUNCIATION AND COMPULSORY COMPREHENSION

Please read the following text aloud, taking your time to pronounce each word carefully. Please use a dictionary and the glossary in appendix A as needed to help you understand the passage. Take your time. This is not a timed exercise, so there is no reason to rush. If you feel yourself becoming fatigued, take a rest and come back to it later.

Frontal lobes: Amongst the many functions of the frontal lobes is the control and management of voluntary movement throughout the body. The sensorimotor cortex, consisting of the motor strip and sensory strip, control willed movements on the side of the body opposite the hemisphere in question (left hemisphere manages the right side of the body). The motor strip sends neural messages to the muscles via a set of pathways and nuclei called the pyramidal system. Voluntary control of motor behavior is modulated by the extrapyramidal system, which is a complex network consisting of the premotor frontal cortex, subcortical gray matter, cerebellum, and vestibular system. Lesions in the pyramidal or extra-pyramidal systems can provoke a variety of speech or language disorders. In front of the motor strip is a portion of frontal lobe called the supplementary motor cortex. This region of the brain plays a critical role for language as it seems to be partially responsible for initiation of motor activity. The ability to initiate spontaneous utterances is impaired by lesions in this region or in the white matter pathways descending from this area to subcortical motor structures. The frontal premotor association cortex is thought to be responsible for synthesizing sensory stimuli coming from throughout the brain and coordinating them with plans of action. Therefore, the frontal lobes mediate abstract thinking, problem solving, and judgment. Damage to this portion of the brain may cause behavioral and personality changes, including impaired judgment, poor strategic planning, and impaired insight, all of which are important for normal language functions.

Temporal lobes: One of the primary functions of the temporal lobes is hearing. Nerve fibers travel from the cranial auditory nerves through the brain stem and thalamus to the auditory cortex in the temporal lobe, making many intermediate connections along the way. Neural impulses from peripheral and central auditory pathways then undergo elaboration and analysis in the auditory association area, located in the posterior portion of the superior temporal gyrus (Wernicke's area). This region is responsible for developing the analysis of auditory stimuli to the point of comprehension. This task is carried out by means of multiple cortical associations, linking auditory stimuli with those from other sensory systems.

Parietal lobes: The primary function of the parietal lobes is perception and elaboration of somesthetic sensations (bodily awareness sensations, including touch, pressure, and position in space). As with motor control in the frontal lobes, somesthesis is organized in the hemisphere opposite the side of the body involved. Somesthetic sensations reach the postcentral gyrus, which is also called the sensory strip. These stimuli travel by means of short association fibers to the secondary sensory association regions located posteriorly in the parietal lobe. The somesthetic sensations are analyzed, elaborated, and connected with multiple stimuli arriving from other parts of the brain. Eventually, an image of one's own body and its position in space emerges. Damage to this part of the brain can produce not only loss of sensation of touch but also impaired recognition of one's own body and a loss of the ability to appreciate spatial concepts.

Occipital lobes: The primary function of the occipital lobes is the processing of vision. The retina of the eye receives visual stimuli and then transmits them via the optic nerve and the thalamus to the primary visual cortex in the occipital lobe. Here the neural impulses are perceived as meaningless flashes of light. To be understood in a meaningful way, the neural information within the visual system must be further analyzed, elaborated, and connected with stimuli from other parts of the brain and from memory systems. This higher-order analysis takes place in the visual association cortex.

Limbic system: The limbic system is a complex network of cortical and subcortical structures that mediates emotion. Major elements of the limbic system include the uncus (part of the olfactory system), parahippocampal gyrus, hippocampus (part of the memory system within the temporal lobes), fornix (major association pathway), mammillary bodies (in the thalamic region), mammillothalamic tract, and cingulate gyrus. Closely linked to the limbic system are the hypothalamus, amygdala, and frontal association cortex. Memories, the desire to produce language, feelings, and the emotional aspect of thought are all mediated by the limbic system. Anatomical systems necessary for cognitive functions, such as language, spatial concepts, understanding of meaning, and so forth, are all linked to the limbic system.

"Zone of language": The zone of language was defined by Dejerine in the early 1900s as that region of the left hemisphere responsible for language. Located within the distribution of the middle cerebral artery, the zone of language surrounds the sylvian fissure on the lateral surface of the hemisphere, incorporating portions of the frontal, parietal, and temporal lobes. Anteriorly, the zone extends to Broca's area (in the premotor region of the frontal lobe). Posteriorly, it extends to Wernicke's area (the auditory association cortex in the posterior portion of the superior temporal gyrus). Connecting Wernicke's and Broca's areas are subcortical white matter pathways, including the arcuate fasciculus and superior longitudinal fasciculus. These white matter pathways pass through the angular gyrus and supramarginal gyrus at the posterior rim of the sylvian fissure, where temporal and parietal lobes come together. These gyri are association areas where many neural interconnections from all over the brain occur. Lesions in different parts of the zone of language may produce different aphasia syndromes. The zone of language should not be considered the "center" for language (that is, a region of the brain where language is located). Rather, it should be regarded as a critical component of several overlapping neural networks, widely distributed throughout the brain, whose total combined activity has the effect of producing language as we know it (Helm-Estabrooks and Albert 1991).

We realize that was difficult, so it may be necessary to take a break. When you are ready, come back to the book and continue with your recovery.

LANGUAGE IN YOUR LIFE

Language is a central part of human life. Some have said that the complexity of the human language is what has separated us from the animals. Language is inherent in almost everything we do. In fact, it is intimately tied to the very way we think.

Most of the cognitive-communication detriments that you suffer from can be overcome through practice. You will, of course, use language every day of your life. If you become consciously aware of this fact and you practice improving your language skills, they will undoubtedly improve. Continue with exercises that are similar to the ones not only in this chapter, but throughout this book. You can pick up puzzle books in almost any store. You can also continue to read challenging texts. Is there an area that you have always wanted to learn about, but never had the time? Pick up a couple of books on it and take the time to understand them. Practice using language, and you will start to heal your mind.

CHAPTER 12

Visuospatial Processing

Good visuospatial skills are essential to your daily living activities. Visuospatial skills include not only your ability to make out and identify particular shapes and objects, but also your ability to place them in space and understand these objects in the context of your greater field of vision. For example, if you were able to see a car and understand what the object was, but were not able to relate it to your greater field of vision and see it driving down the road, this would be a pretty big problem. Visuospatial processing problems are often a result of an MTBI. Because human beings are such visual creatures, the very way that we orient ourselves and operate in the world is largely based on the way that we see. For this reason, visuospatial difficulties often manifest themselves as difficulties with functional mobility, reading, comprehension, attention, concentration, memory, headaches, photophobia (sensitivity to light), and field loss (places in your line of sight that seem blank or missing) for people who have suffered an MTBI.

According to Dr. Allen Cohen, visual problems arising from trauma that affect the functional visual system can be identified as post-trauma vision syndrome (PTVS). PTVS symptoms may include tendency for the eyes to turn out, difficulty focusing on a target, poor eye movement, double or blurred near vision, perceived movement of print, eye muscle weakness, headaches, and sensitivity to light. These characteristics can be treated effectively through neurorehabilitation, lens prescriptions, and prism lenses (Cohen 2003).

If you have been able to read and understand this book up to this point, it is likely that your visuospatial processing skills are in fairly good shape. However, it is possible that certain areas of this processing mechanism have been affected. It is therefore valuable for you to study this chapter, assess where your weaknesses might lie, and learn some strategies that you can use to overcome these problems.

THE WAY THAT VISION WORKS

As you learned in chapter 8, the cornea, lens, and iris work together to send an image to the retina at the back of the eye. The image focuses on the retina and stimulates photoreceptors, rods and cones, which turn light stimulus into electrical signals. The electrical signals travel directly to the brain along the optic nerve, which ends in the thalamus and the brain stem. From here, the fibers extend to the visual areas of the cerebral cortex in the occipital and parietal lobes. The brain is the real processor of vision. The eyes are only the initial receptor.

What follows is a fairly technical description of the way that vision works. Please read it slowly and carefully if you are having problems understanding any part of it. Don't be afraid to use the dictionary and the glossary of this book if you need to. This is important information for you to have a basic understanding of if you are to recover your visuospatial processing skills. Think of the following text as another exercise in compulsory comprehension, like the one we did in chapter 11. Take your time, read carefully, and rest as you need to.

Where Vision Is Processed

The occipital lobe (in the back of the skull) contains the visual cortex. It recognizes and identifies visual information and allows you to decide how to use the visual information. The frontal eye fields anticipate where things should be and direct the eyes to the appropriate location. The parietal lobe focuses on objects and their relationship to one another. The ability to process spatial information is controlled by the ventral visual stream, which is essentially neurocircuitry that connects the occipital, parietal, and frontal lobes. The temporal lobe focuses on color, form, detail, and size to accurately identify objects, and assigns emotional relevance to events. The circuitry that controls these functions is called the dorsal visual stream and it connects the occipital, temporal, and frontal regions. Objects with strong motivational relevance get more representation. There are also hemispheric differences with visual processing. The left hemisphere processes limited objects one at a time in an orderly fashion, which is necessary for reading. The right hemisphere processes visual information more globally, categorizing information in groups (Hamby 2000; Tortora and Grabowski 1993).

Visual signals in the visual pathway are processed by at least three separate systems in the brain. One system processes information related to the shape of objects, the second is related to the color of objects, and the third processes information about movement, location, and spatial organization (Tortora and Grabowski 1993).

Visual Skills Hierarchy

The skills that you require in order to process visual information in the way described above can also be broken down into different components and tasks. By examining and assessing your visual skills in this way, you will get a better grasp on where you might have visual deficits and how you might be able to overcome these problem areas. Each of these sets of tasks actually build, one on top of the other, in order to form a hierarchy. We have talked throughout this book about the hierarchical nature of cognitive function. This is just another area where this concept holds true.

If you are having problems in the lower, or foundational, levels of the hierarchy, it is likely that you will notice problems in your visual processing skills in every other part of this complex system. Let's take a look at how this visual hierarchy works, and what different skills make up each of its three levels.

Tier One

Visuospatial skills are hierarchical in nature. The foundation of visual skills includes:

- control of eye movement

- visual fields (the whole area that the eyes can see)

- visual acuity (the ability to see clearly)

Control of eye movement: Ninety-five percent of individuals with brain injury have impaired eye movement that is not due to cranial nerve damage. Eye movement keeps the visual image steady and focused. The eyes must work together to see just one image and provide depth perception. Eye muscle imbalances may cause a strain on the eye, possible headaches, squinting, double vision, and agitation.

Visual fields impact the amount of visual information that can be observed. Visual field deficits due to MTBI result in an increased number of upper vision losses, which significantly impact driving. Individuals with visual field deficits are generally unaware of their deficit. An MTBI can impact any portion of the visual field.

Visual acuity affects the quality of visual information. Impaired visual acuity may show up as blurriness, difficulty with reading or walking, reaching and grasping difficulties, headaches, and agitation.

It is not very likely that you are having problems with these visuospatial processing skills. If you were, it would be unlikely that you would be able to read this book.

Tier Two

The next tier of the visual skills hierarchy includes visual attention, scanning, and pattern recognition.

Scanning is a motor skill that entails movement of the eyes. An organized search is known as a scan path. The most common problem with scanning is neglect, which is a visual attention disorder.

Visual attention is necessary for scanning. If visual attention is decreased, visual scanning will be difficult because eye movements are slower and less smooth. Following an MTBI that involves the frontal eye fields, scanning becomes disorganized and random, as the eyes have trouble anticipating where they should be directed.

Pattern recognition is the ability to identify the form and details of an object. Hemispheric differences are noted in pattern recognition. The left hemisphere is better able to process detail with greater frequency and contrast, with examples such as quilting, reading, games, and numbers. The right hemisphere is better able to process information of low contrast and frequency, and with greater distortions such as whole forms and complete pictures, like the view outside a window.

There are two pathways that organize this tier of visual processing (Cohen 2003). The first pathway is the *focal pathway* or *central vision*, which allows you to see details of a single object in your environment. This is learned and based on experience and culture. An example of the focal pathway would be locating the cream of mushroom soup in the soup section of the grocery store.

The second pathway is the *ambient pathway*. It is the visual process that obtains visual information from peripheral vision. It detects information regarding events and where you are in space to help you with balance, movement, coordination, and posture. An example of the ambient pathway would be locating the soup section in the grocery store.

The focal pathway provides information regarding what is seen and the ambient pathway provides information about where one is in space and where one is looking. Both pathways must work together for the visual system to be efficient. The pathway typically impacted by an MTBI is the ambient pathway or our ability to process spatial information. Before moving on, let's do an exercise that utilizes both pathways.

EXERCISE: BLOCK DECIPHER

The large design on the next page is made up of the individual blocks below. The blocks can be turned any direction and can be used several times. In the grid below, write the number of the block that corresponds to that position in the overall design.

1	2	3	4	5

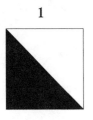  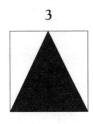 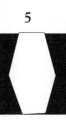 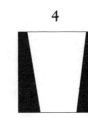

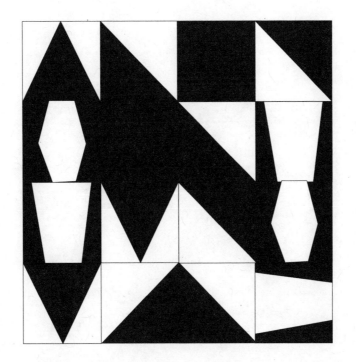

Check appendix C for the answers. If you had problems completing this exercise, or got less than half of the answers correct, then it is likely that you are having problems with this area of visual processing. Later in the chapter, there will be further assessments for this potential problem and some things you can do to overcome it.

Tier Three

The final tier of the visual hierarchy includes visual memory and visual cognition.

Visual memory is the ability to recognize and identify objects and discriminate between objects depending on previous visual memory.

Visual cognition is the ability to mentally manipulate and organize visual information. It is a learned skill that comes from intelligence and experience. Visual cognition is the highest skill in the visual system.

The following exercise will help you understand whether or not you are having difficulties in this tier of visuospatial processing.

EXERCISE: VISUAL DISCRIMINATION

Choose from the four figures below the one that is the same as the figure in the box.

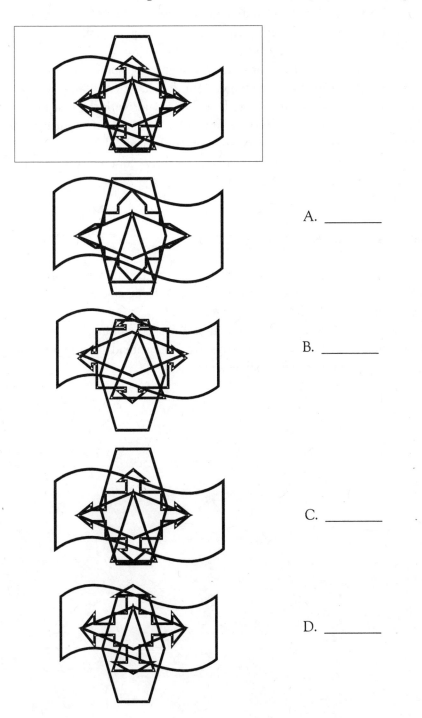

A. _____

B. _____

C. _____

D. _____

Check your answer in appendix C. If you have problems identifying the figure, then it is likely that you are having some problems with visual discrimination, which is a tier-three visuospatial processing component.

REPAIRING YOUR VISUOSPATIAL DEFICITS

In the exercises above, you were given the opportunity to get a grasp on where your problems in this area of cognitive functioning may lie. If you were to go to a neuro-ophthalmologist for a full assessment of your visuospatial processing dysfunction, they would give you a set of exercises that are quite similar in nature to the ones that we have given you here.

Now that you have a grip on what may be going wrong for you, we will give you some exercises and ideas about how you can start to improve your situation and overcome your deficits.

As we stated earlier in the chapter, it is unlikely that you are having problems with the first tier of visuospatial processing functions, because you would have a hard time reading this book. If you fear that you are in fact having problems in this area, you should seek professional neurological help.

Based on this, our overview of how you can repair this part of your cognitive function will revolve around the upper two levels in the visuospatial processing hierarchy.

Visual Attention, Scanning, and Pattern Recognition

Your skills in these areas need to be exercised in two different realms: the two-dimensional realm and the three-dimensional realm. Obviously, it takes a lot more mental energy to be able to successfully scan and recognize patterns in the three-dimensional realm.

The easiest way for you to get started with repairing your visual attention, scanning, and pattern recognition skills is through a set of simple exercises. The following exercises should be a good start toward retraining these parts of your visuospatial processing mechanisms.

EXERCISE: LOCATE THE REGIONS OF THE BRAIN

Below are sections of the brain from the picture of the brain at the bottom of the page. With a pen, circle the regions on the whole brain that are represented by the sections shown directly below.

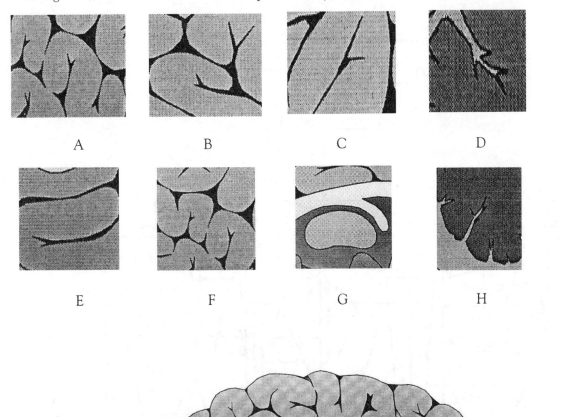

A   B   C   D

E   F   G   H

Check appendix C for the answers. If you had problems with this exercise, don't worry—there are some ways that we can help you improve in these areas. Before learning some tips, try one more exercise.

EXERCISE: FIGURE GROUND

Circle the following figure each time it appears in the picture below. There are three occurrences. Time yourself for this exercise and enter your time below in seconds. Check appendix C for the answers.

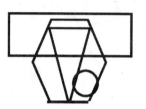

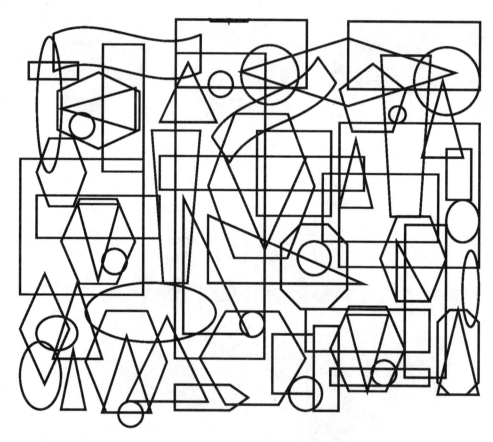

Time: _____ seconds

Review your performance above and compare your time to the times indicated below.

20 seconds or less = above average

21–45 seconds = average

46–72 seconds = below average

73 seconds or more = impairment

This exercise is built not only to test and help repair your abilities to effectively scan and recognize patterns, but also to test your visual processing speed. If you feel like you sometimes have a harder time recognizing patterns than you used to, it is likely that your visual processing speed has slowed some. This is very natural for people who have an MTBI. With time and practice, it will improve.

Retraining Your Scan Path

One of the most important ways that you can improve the skills that you are working on in the exercises above is to do what is called *retraining your scan path*. Your scan path is everything that comes into your line of vision as you look over or scan across any type of visual stimuli. Following an MTBI, the scan path tends to become random and impulsive. That is, you have a harder time looking over information in an orderly and organized fashion. Sometimes this is because the movement of your eyes has become erratic and sometimes it is because your visuospatial processing centers have been damaged and have "forgotten" how to analyze information in an orderly fashion. In order to retrain your scan path, there are three simple steps you need to employ:

- Utilize your finger as a search guide.

- Keep your gaze on that finger.

- Organize your search by starting at one point and systematically scanning horizontally to the next boundary in a limited space.

Try it. Go back through the exercises above and see if you find it easier to scan the material using the strategies above to retrain your scan path.

Over time, your eyes and brain will heal and you will not have to continue to use your finger in the way described above. But to facilitate this healing process, it is a good idea to use this technique.

You can continue to work on your two-dimensional scanning abilities at home. There are many puzzle books, board games, and video games that utilize these skills. The Where's Waldo books, and pattern searches like the ones found earlier in this book, can help you to retrain your visual scanning and pattern recognition abilities. In addition, practical living skills like reading bus schedules, reading a map, or looking up numbers in a phone book really revolve around these visuospatial processing abilities.

Taking It to the Third Dimension

It is one thing to be able to pick out patterns in a puzzle, but it is something else entirely to use these skills in your day-to-day life. Nonetheless, visual scanning and pattern recognition are skills that you use every day to understand and interpret your world. Take these skills to the world outside and practice them.

If you want a challenge, try going grocery shopping at the busiest time of the day. When you are in the grocery store, your visual scanning and pattern recognition skills are put to the test in a three-dimensional field. Not only do you have to scan the aisles to figure out where certain sections of the grocery store are, you have to scan those sections to find the products that you need. Going to the store when it is busy adds a level of distraction that will force you to exercise that part of your mind a bit more.

Activities like these will not only help you recover your visuospatial processing capabilities, they will help you take your recovery with you to the world outside.

Visual Memory and Visual Cognition

As stated earlier in the chapter, visual memory and visual cognition are the highest skills in the visuospatial hierarchy. In fact, these two skills are really the culmination of all the other skills listed, and allow us to do things that take a very complex set of visual processing skills. Things like driving a car, fixing a flat tire, or moving a large desk out of a room with a small door require the use of these tier-three skills.

It may not be entirely obvious to you what the difference is between visual memory and pattern recognition. The real difference here lies in cognition. Pattern recognition is simply your ability to see and associate a particular pattern with another that is similar to it. This skill does not require you to think about this memorized pattern and apply it to other aspects of your life. Visual memory is, in fact, much more complicated than simple pattern recognition. Visual memory actually requires that you apply what you have learned to a particular circumstance. Perhaps you have driven around a town that is a bit unfamiliar to you and been lost. As you drive, you slowly start to realize that you have seen the places that you are driving past before. As you continue to explore the town, a pattern starts to emerge in your mind and soon enough you remember where the streets are and where you should turn to get to where you want to go. This is visual memory. Your tier-two visuospatial skills would not be capable of processing this type of information on their own.

As you might guess, the best way to recover these skills is practice. You could start off on the two-dimensional level like we did for the earlier skills. Simple memory card games are a very good way to start exercising this part of your mind. Try the game where you place all the cards face down in rows. Turn over two cards at a time until you've matched all the cards into pairs.

As you get more accustomed to using these skills, you can accelerate your learning process by involving yourself in skills that require even more sophisticated use of visual cognition and visual memory. Try walking into a mall that you are not particularly familiar with and walking back out using the same path that you entered by. This will test your visual memory and cognition skills on a much higher level than the memory card games.

YOUR SIGHT, YOUR WORLD

The way that you see affects the way that you live in the world. As with all of the other components of your cognitive function, visuospatial processing influences not only how you see, but the very way that you think.

By practicing the exercises given in this chapter and taking them with you into the world, you will start to see an improvement in your visuospatial processing capabilities. Though you may have problems in this area now, soon enough you will recover from your deficits and see the world again.

This chapter completes the cognitive portion of this workbook. The remainder of the book will help you overcome mood problems you may be encountering due to your condition.

CHAPTER 13

Depression

In this chapter, we are going to examine depression. Depression is the single most common psychiatric disorder associated with brain injury. We will take a look at its causes and help you to gain a better understanding of its dynamics. We will discuss depression within the context of recovery from your injury and the changes you might currently be experiencing due to depression. I will guide you through the process of ascertaining if you might be depressed and help you to find the appropriate care. Please be aware that a full treatment program for depression is well beyond the scope of this chapter. This chapter will focus primarily on helping you to know if depression is a problem for you and how it may be contributing to the symptoms of your MTBI. If you are suffering from depression, you may need to seek professional psychological help. There are also many good books on the market that deal specifically with this problem. Two of these are *The Depression Workbook* and *Your Depression Map*, both of which are published by New Harbinger Publications.

DEPRESSION AND MTBI ARE INTERTWINED

Often it is difficult to differentiate depression from other symptoms related to brain injury. For instance, the following characteristics are associated with depression:

■   Sleep disturbances

- Changes in appetite

- Fatigue

- Apathy

- Self-loathing

- Lack of sexual desire (decreased libido)

- Inability to feel pleasure (anhedonia)

- Lack of motivation

- Thoughts of suicide

- Feelings of hopelessness

- Feelings of helplessness

Nearly all of these symptoms are also side effects of an MTBI. To further complicate matters, depression and MTBI symptoms combine to create a cycle where depressive symptoms exacerbate MTBI symptoms (difficulty concentrating, memory deficits, sleep disturbances, fatigue) and these heightened symptoms then deepen the depression.

The Differences between Depression and MTBI

There are many similarities between depression and MTBI, as described above. Nonetheless, it is important to remember that while your depression may be intimately linked with your MTBI (in fact, it may even have been caused by the neurochemical changes that occurred when you were injured), it is a separate condition that can be diagnosed independently of your head trauma. According to the *Quick Reference to the Diagnostic Criteria from Diagnostic and Statistical Manual of Mental Disorders* (American Psychiatric Association 1994), a major depression is defined as five or more of the following symptoms that last for two consecutive weeks with symptoms present nearly every day for most of the day. One of these symptoms must be depressed mood or a general loss of interest and pleasure.

1. Depressed mood most of the day (feels sad or empty)

2. Markedly diminished interest or pleasure in activities

3. Change in appetite or significant weight gain or loss (5 percent of body weight in one month)

4. Sleep disturbance (insomnia or hypersomnia)

5. Significantly increased or decreased activity level

6. Fatigue or loss of energy

7. Excessive guilt or feelings of worthlessness

8. Poor concentration or indecisiveness

9. Recurrent thoughts of death or suicide

If you feel that this description applies to you, you should seriously consider obtaining professional help. While depression can be cured in other ways, professional help is really your fastest route to a full recovery.

The following questionnaire should give you a better idea as to whether or not you are suffering from clinical depression.

EXERCISE: DEPRESSION ASSESSMENT

This assessment is modified from a geriatric depression scale (Sheikh et al. 1991; Yesavage et al. 1983; Brink et al. 1982). Answer the questions by circling yes or no.

1. Do you feel dissatisfied with your life?	Yes / No
2. Have you dropped many of your activities and interests?	Yes / No
3. Do you feel that your life is empty?	Yes / No
4. Do you often get bored?	Yes / No
5. Do you feel your future is hopeless?	Yes / No
6. Are you bothered by thoughts that you can't get out of your head?	Yes / No
7. Are you down and in poor spirits most of the time?	Yes / No
8. Are you afraid something bad is going to happen to you?	Yes / No
9. Do you feel sad most of the time?	Yes / No
10. Do you often feel helpless?	Yes / No
11. Do you often get restless and fidgety?	Yes / No
12. Do you prefer to stay home rather than go out and do new things?	Yes / No
13. Do you frequently worry about the future?	Yes / No
14. Do you feel you have more problems with memory than most?	Yes / No

15. Do you think it is difficult and draining to be alive now?   Yes / No

16. Do you often feel downhearted and blue?   Yes / No

17. Do you feel pretty worthless the way you are now?   Yes / No

18. Do you worry a lot about the past?   Yes / No

19. Do you feel life is dull and boring?   Yes / No

20. Is it hard for you to get a start on new projects?   Yes / No

21. Are you lacking energy?   Yes / No

22. Do you feel that your situation is hopeless?   Yes / No

23. Do you feel that most people are better off than you are?   Yes / No

24. Do you frequently get upset about little things?   Yes / No

25. Do you frequently feel like crying?   Yes / No

26. Do you have trouble concentrating?   Yes / No

27. Do you have trouble getting up in the morning?   Yes / No

28. Do you prefer to avoid social gatherings?   Yes / No

29. Is it difficult for you to make decisions?   Yes / No

30. Is your mind less clear than it used to be?   Yes / No

Count the number of times that you answered yes to the above questions and put the number in the space provided.

Total number of yes answers: _____

If you answered yes to ten or more of the questions above, then it is likely that you have depression. Please remember that this questionnaire should not take the place of a complete psychiatric evaluation. However, this assessment, in conjunction with the information from the DSM-IV, should give you a pretty good idea as to whether or not you are actually suffering from depression.

THE PROBLEM OF DEPRESSION AND MTBI

Depression is a very difficult condition to face and overcome by itself. It presents a special problem when it is diagnosed in conjunction with MTBI. As was stated earlier, when you are suffering from both MTBI and depression, a vicious cycle can be created wherein your depression deepens your MTBI symptoms, which in turn enhances your depression.

As I have said several times in this chapter, your best course of action to overcome this problem is to seek professional help (there will be more on this in a bit). However, there are a few strategies that you can employ right now that will help you cope with your depression until you are able to find a psychiatrist.

Exercise

It has been proven again and again, throughout the literature on depression, that exercise is directly related to your mood. If you are not already working out, the easiest and fastest way that you can start to cope with your depression is to engage in some sort of regular exercise routine. This doesn't have to be anything complicated or demanding. Simply pick a physical activity that you enjoy (or think you may enjoy) and start doing it. Something as simple as going for a walk or a run can really help you cope with your depressed feelings. Activities like these also have the added benefit of getting you out of the house and into the world.

Before starting any kind of strenuous exercise routine, I would highly recommend that you consult with your physician. Remember that your brain may still be tender after the injury, and there may be certain types of exercise you need to stay away from. Don't let that discourage you. I am sure that with your doctor's help, you can come up with some kind of physical activity that you can engage in.

Socialize

Being around and talking with other people can be very helpful if you are depressed. Now that you have suffered from an MTBI, you may feel very isolated and alone. It may be that you feel people don't really understand your condition and what is going on for you. However, if you aren't communicating with and communing with others, this feeling will only increase.

There is an endless array of things that you can do with the people in your life. Why don't you ask a friend to go to the movies with you? Try asking your sister if she wants to go have dinner and a chat. What about that old friend you haven't spoken with in years? Give them a call. Even if you don't think you feel up to it, or you are worried about how people might react, give it a shot. I would almost guarantee that you will get a different reaction than you expect.

Another component of personal interactions is being open with the way that you feel. Simply talking about your depression and the concerns you have with your MTBI can be immensely therapeutic. You shouldn't rely on this to "heal" you. However, I am sure that you have a friend or family member who would be more than happy to hear about your worries and concerns and discuss them with you. You never know—they may have some kind words or good advice that can help.

Counter Negative Thoughts

Countering your negative thoughts is one of the centerpieces of a cognitive behavioral therapy (CBT) treatment course for depression. If you choose to see a therapist who specializes in CBT, you will very likely get a more complete description of what this process is about.

Countering your negative thoughts is really a three-step process that consists of monitoring your thoughts, employing the "downward arrow," and reassessing the truth of these thoughts. Let's go through each step one at a time.

Monitor Your Thoughts

When you are depressed, it is often difficult to get a grip on what is making you depressed. You may be in a generally crappy mood and think that you are feeling bad for no reason. It also may seem that at times during your day this bad mood becomes even worse for no apparent reason.

One of the key factors in depression is *negative thinking*. Negative thinking happens when you make the worst out of any situation. For example, you may think, "I will never get better after this MTBI." Such thoughts can really drive your depression.

In order to get a better grip on such thoughts, I would suggest that you keep track of all the times during the day when you feel a shift in your mood. Try doing this for about two weeks. Carry a notebook around with you, and every time your mood drops, ask yourself, "What was I thinking about right then?" Really try to work out what the thought was that made you feel bad. Once you have a good idea of what thought is making you feel bad, write it down. Try to do this every time you feel a drop in your mood. In two weeks, you will have a very thorough list of the thoughts that are driving your depression.

Here is an example to illustrate the process I am talking about.

David was having a really hard time figuring out how to access information on the shared computer drive at his office. He knew that his computer was networked to all of the others in the building, but he just couldn't get the sales data he was looking for.

He asked the coworker who sat at the desk next to his for some help. In what seemed like a split second his coworker had all of the information up on his screen. This made David feel lousy, but he couldn't quite figure out why at first. He put some thought to it and he realized that when she had gotten the information so quickly, he thought, "Now that I have a brain injury, I will never be able to work that fast again." As you can imagine, this idea caused him to feel terrible. He took note of the thought and wrote it down in the thought record he had been keeping.

EXERCISE: THE DOWNWARD ARROW

In many cases, the first thought that you have is not the only thought that you have. Underlying your *automatic thoughts* (thoughts that pop up automatically in a situation) are deeper general beliefs about yourself and the world around you. In order to gain access to these *core beliefs*, psychologists often employ what is called the *downward arrow method*. This method is really fairly simple. First take your automatic thought and write it down. Why don't you take one of your automatic thoughts and write it in the space below? (This exercise has been adapted from *Your Depression Map* by Randy Paterson.)

_____

This thought may or may not be true. For the moment, let's assume that it is absolutely true. If this were the case, what would it mean about you? Write your answer below.

_____

And if this were true, what would it mean? What would the consequence be?

_____

And if this were true. . . ?

_____

Continue this process until you can't think of any other associated thoughts or consequences. Once you have come to this point, you will likely have found a thought or thought pattern that you hold as a core belief. Let's follow through with the example of David to get a better feel for this process.

David had the thought, "I will never get better after this MTBI." But he wanted to know more about what was affecting him and making him feel depressed, so he decided to employ the downward arrow method. This was the train of thoughts that he came up with:

"If I can't get better from my accident, I will lose my job and my friends."

"If I lose my job and my friends, I will just stay at home and stop trying to get better."

"If I don't try to get better, my mind will get weaker and weaker, and soon I won't be able to function at all."

"If I can't function, nobody will help me and I will die alone."

"My life is now hopeless."

Reassessing Your Thoughts, or Learning to Tell the Truth

As you might imagine, if David came to the conclusions that his friends would leave him, he would die alone, and that his life was hopeless, this could contribute very significantly to his depression.

What if, on the other hand, he was able to tell himself, "I wish this MTBI had never happened, but I can get better and I will soon be able to do this job much better." This would very likely make him feel much better than the thought, "I will never get better after this MTBI." The ironic thing is that the statement that he can get better is the one that is really true!

The truth about automatic thoughts is that at best they are enormous exaggerations and at worst they are downright lies. This kind of catastrophic thinking is not only terribly unrealistic, it does nothing to help your situation.

In order to combat your unrealistic automatic thoughts, try being more realistic about the situation. Make a real assessment of what is happening for you. Let's try it. Write your automatic thought on the line below.

_____

Now step back from your thinking and read your statement objectively. Is it really the truth? How could you state it more realistically? Write your revised thought on the line below.

_____

You will likely notice that the new thought is much more moderate. This is almost always the case. Normally the reality of a situation is much less extreme than we make it out to be.

Take this new thought with you. Remember it, and every time you have a negative automatic thought, try replacing it with this new thought. At first this might seem difficult, or even untrue. It is a funny thing with humans that we tend to believe outrageous exaggerations more easily than the truth. However, over time you will start to realize that this new thought is much closer to the truth than your old exaggerated way of thinking.

Perhaps you, like David, think that you will never recover from your MTBI and this thought is making you depressed. But really the thought isn't true at all. It is a shame that the MTBI happened, but you can get better. The very fact that you are working on the exercises in this book is something that you should be proud of. This book is leading you toward recovery even as you read this sentence. Try to keep this in mind.

SEEKING PROFESSIONAL HELP

There is a vast world of professional psychiatric help that is available to you. I can't stress enough how much difference seeing a therapist can make in terms of recovering from depression. If you even have the slightest sense that you are depressed, you should see a therapist.

Having said that, there are a few things you should keep in mind when looking for a person to help you overcome depression.

Who Should You See?

These days there is an almost endless array of different therapeutic modalities and different types of therapists to choose from. I simply don't have the space here to go through and talk about all of them. Nonetheless, there are some things to keep in mind when choosing a therapist.

It is important that you find someone who is familiar with MTBI if that is at all possible. Because MTBI contributes to depression in very particular ways, it is important that your therapist has an understanding of your condition and what it means. You may want to see a neuropsychologist, as these practitioners are more likely to understand the ways in which neurological impairments affect moods. The easiest way to tell if the person you are thinking of seeing is familiar with MTBI is to ask. When you are setting up your first appointment, simply ask the receptionist if this doctor is acquainted with MTBI. It is also a good idea to address this issue directly with the therapist in your first session.

Therapy Is for You

Always keep in mind that therapy is about you. This is a vital part of your recovery. It is important that you give a therapist a good chance, but if you don't feel comfortable with the person, or you are afraid that they don't really have a grip on your condition, there is absolutely no reason for you to stay with them. Make sure that you are comfortable with your therapist. If you shortchange yourself, you are shortchanging your recovery. Keep yourself in mind when you are selecting a therapist.

Be Open and Ask Questions

The more open and honest you are in therapy, the more you will get out of it. It is often difficult to express your innermost feelings with other people. This is why it is so vitally important that you find a therapist whom you can trust. Try to be open during the therapy process and share your true fears and worries with your therapist.

Never be afraid to ask questions. Your therapist is a psychological professional who is there to help you. If there are questions that you want to ask or specific concerns that you have, you should always feel free to bring them up. Information is power. The more you find out about yourself, the better position you will be in to help yourself. And sometimes the only way to learn is to ask.

A Word on Medications

There are many psychiatric medications available to help you overcome depression. It may be that your therapist refers you to a psychiatrist to see whether or not medications would be helpful for you. It may very well be that they are. However, if you are already on medications, you need to make sure to communicate this information to your psychiatrist. In addition, as was mentioned earlier in the book, all of the medications that you consider taking should be approved by the doctor whom you have chosen to manage your health care. There are many important considerations when dealing with these types of medications. Antidepressants can have some very serious side effects when interacting with other drugs. It behooves you to make sure you have all the necessary information before starting a regimen of psychiatric medicine.

A WORD OF REASSURANCE

Hope. That is the word of reassurance I would like you to keep in mind. Hope. There is always hope. You can get better. Your depression can improve, and your MTBI symptoms can be decreased, as we have demonstrated throughout this book. Try to hang on to hope. It is often difficult, but it is always there.

Since your MTBI, you are likely dealing with some very serious physical, mental, and psychological concerns. You may even be questioning some of the deepest parts of yourself, wondering what you are worth and why you are alive. Please remember that each person has a place in this world. If you apply yourself, you will get better. And your place in this world will be revealed to you.

CHAPTER 14

Anxiety

Anxiety is very often a side effect or a direct result of an MTBI. It may be that the trauma to your brain has affected your neurochemistry, making you more susceptible to feelings of anxiety. It also may be that you tend to feel anxious when you try to focus and can't or when you try to remember something and have a hard time with it. You may even have become more sensitive to light and sound, which can lead to feelings of anxiety. For whatever reasons, anxiety is often a problem for people who have had an MTBI.

THE NATURE OF ANXIETY

Anxiety is a physiological state. That is, it has both physical and psychological components. In fact, anxiety is a complex set of physiological responses that happen in our minds and bodies for a number of reasons. It may be that you have heard of the *fight-or-flight response*.

When our ancestors were in danger, their nervous system automatically prepared them to fight the danger or run away from it. In order to do this, a heightened state is induced in the body and mind that includes the release of a vast amount of adrenaline into the blood. This heightened state of arousal is what allowed ancient people to successfully negotiate life-threatening situations on a regular basis. In the modern era, we are not faced with the same frequency and type of life-or-death situations that our predecessors had to deal with so many years ago. Unfortunately, our physiological evolution has not kept up with the advances of society, and our bodies are still programmed to react in this very severe manner whenever we perceive that we are in danger, even if that danger is not at all life-threatening. This is the very nature of anxiety. You perceive that you are in some kind of danger and your body and mind automatically respond with a set of preprogrammed physiological responses. Because this danger is only perceived and we have no reason to either fight or flee in most situations, we are left with a feeling of anxiety.

The antithesis of anxiety is relaxation. It has often been said that anxiety cannot exist in a relaxed body. This is, in fact, true. As such, this chapter will focus on teaching you how to fully relax. When you learn to truly relax, you will be able to institute relaxation when you start to feel anxious. But before moving on to specific relaxation exercises, let's have a look at how MTBI and anxiety affect one another.

ANXIETY AND MTBI

Much like depression, anxiety and MTBI symptoms can have an adverse affect on one another. Often a vicious cycle is created (much as it is when you are depressed) when you are having troubles with both anxiety and MTBI. Well-controlled studies have shown that anxiety and stress impair attention, resulting in diminished memory and cognition. That means that the more anxious you are, the more likely it will be that your cognitive function is impaired in some way. If you start to feel anxious because you are having problems with your memory, for example, your anxiety will make it even more difficult for you to remember. This may make you feel more anxious, which will make it even more difficult to remember, and so the cycle begins.

The good news is that there is a way out of this cycle. The answer is relaxation. So let's starting teaching you how to relax.

RELAXATION

Relaxing is far more than simply chilling out on the couch. It is very likely that you have no idea what it feels like to be completely relaxed. In our fast-paced technological society, most of us have never really been taught how to relax completely. To be relaxed is to enter into a state of deep physiological peace. Your body is at ease and your mind is at rest. Just as it has been proven that anxiety interrupts good cognitive function, there are many studies that have shown that relaxation not only improves cognition, but improves your overall mental and physical health.

There are many relaxation exercises to choose from. I will teach you three that have proven useful for people that have MTBI: deep breathing, progressive muscle relaxation, and visualization. Before learning the actual techniques, you need to learn what it is like to be relaxed.

Learning What Relaxation Feels Like

Because you have likely never been taught to relax, the first step in this process is to learn the difference between feeling tense and feeling relaxed. I could try to describe this difference all day long, but a direct visceral experience of this difference will take you a lot further toward understanding.

EXERCISE: LEARNING TO RELAX

This exercise will help you to differentiate between relaxation and tension. It is vital that you understand and are able to differentiate between being relaxed and being anxious, as deactivation of the fight-or-flight response is essential in your healing process. In just a few minutes, you will become aware of how it feels to be tense. The differences may be subtle for some of these exercises, but the effects are cumulative. Never underestimate the potential of discomfort to distract you. As you compare each part of your body, you may want to rate the relaxed and tensed feeling on a scale of 1 to 10 (with 1 being completely relaxed and 10 being very tense). For example, rank from 1 to 10 what your hands feel like clenched and then unclenched.

For this exercise, sit in an upright chair and place your body in each of the following positions, holding each one for twenty seconds. We will start off with the unrelaxed position so that you can compare the difference in tension within your body and ultimately end up in an overall relaxed state. As you progress through each stage, relax the parts of your body that were previously tense. Take the time necessary to appreciate the difference between relaxed and tense. Do not perform this exercise on areas that have sustained damage or that are injured (for example, if you have back or neck pain, skip those areas).

- **Feet**
  Tense: Place the balls of your feel directly on the floor and lift your heels off the floor.
  Relaxed: Place your feet flat on the floor with your toes spread evenly and the weight distributed evenly between the balls of your feet and your heels.

- **Legs**
  Tense: Cross your legs at the knee and tense the muscles in your calves.
  Relaxed: Place your legs with your feet flat on the floor with ninety-degree angles at the knees and ankles.

- **Back, chest, and stomach**
  Tense: Arch your back and push your stomach forward. Tighten all the muscles in the front and rear of your torso.
  Relaxed: Rest your back gently against the back of your chair. Allow all of the muscles in your back, chest, and stomach to completely relax.

- **Shoulders**
  Tense: Shrug and tense your shoulders and hold them as high as you can get them for twenty seconds.
  Relaxed: Rest your arms on the chair's armrests or place your hands on your upper thighs. Point your fingers inward and keep your elbows slightly bent. Let your shoulders feel broad and firm. Let all of the muscles in your shoulders and neck completely relax.

- **Arms**
  Tense: Stretch your arms straight out in front of you, holding them parallel to the floor. Tighten your forearms, biceps, and triceps. Hold this position for twenty seconds. Feel the tension building in your arms.
  Relaxed: Bend your arms at the elbow with your wrists resting on your thighs. Allow all the muscles in your arms to relax.

- **Hands**
  Tense: Clench your hands into fists and hold for twenty seconds.
  Relaxed: Rest your hands in your lap with the fingers slightly curled, allowing all the small tendons and muscles to completely relax.

- **Neck, jaw, and face**
  Tense: Place your teeth firmly together and slightly flex your jaw muscle. Tuck your chin into your neck and pucker your lips and crinkle your forehead.
  Relaxed: Allow your teeth and lips to part slightly and allow the tension to leave your jaw. Allow the weight of your head to lean slightly forward. Allow all of the muscles in your face to completely relax.

Did you feel a difference between being relaxed and being tense? Try to keep this feeling in mind as you work through the rest of the relaxation exercises in this chapter.

Progressive Muscle Relaxation (PMR)

This technique was first developed by Edmund Jacobson in 1929 and has become one of the cornerstones for anxiety treatment since that time. The basic premise of the exercise is fairly simple: anxiety causes muscle tension, so if you relax the tension in the muscles the anxiety will disappear. This simple concept actually has profound implications for the mind and body. By practicing progressive muscle relaxation, you will have an incredible impact on your anxiety. Before we get started with the actual exercise, there are a few things you should keep in mind as you do this exercise. The following suggestions and the progressive muscle relaxation exercise itself have been adapted from *Coping with Anxiety* by Edmund Bourne and Lorna Garano (2003).

Practice regularly. Going through an entire PMR exercise will take you about twenty minutes. It is important that you set aside the time you need to complete the entire exercise. It is best if you are able to practice this method twice a day. Of course, if this is impossible, then once a day will do. However, I would recommend you do this exercise regularly, not just "whenever you feel like it." To get the most out of any relaxation technique, you need to practice every day and you need to practice at regular times. If you are going to try to do this twice a day, I would recommend doing it upon waking and just before you go to bed. If you can't make this schedule work, then any other regular schedule should serve you well.

Find a quiet place and assume a comfortable position. It is important that you are not interrupted while doing the exercise. Turn off your phones and other things that might distract you. If you invest effort into focusing on the exercise, you will get a lot out of it.

It is also important that you get yourself into a comfortable position. Make sure that your entire body is supported (including your neck and head) as you begin the exercise. Lying on the sofa or a bed with your head on a pillow should do nicely.

Don't worry about anything, including how well you are doing. It is important that you try to put aside your daily worries when you start the exercise. The more you invest in really trying to let your worries pass, the more likely it is you will enter a deeply relaxed state.

Though it is often very difficult, it is also necessary that you not worry about how well you are doing with the exercise. This kind of anxiety can only diminish the effectiveness of PMR. Don't get wrapped up in how well you are doing. Simply do your best and let the exercise happen.

Tense, don't strain. As you go through the exercise, you will be asked to tense and relax various groups of muscles. Make sure that you do not strain the muscles. Tense them naturally and then let go. This is especially true of any areas of your body that have been or are injured due to your accident. If you are at all concerned about certain areas of your body (especially your neck and head), simply skip the part of the exercise that is associated with that part of your body.

Now let's get going with some progressive muscle relaxation.

EXERCISE: PROGRESSIVE MUSCLE RELAXATION

Once you are comfortably supported in a quiet place, follow the steps below:

1. To begin, take three deep abdominal breaths, exhaling slowly each time. As you exhale, imagine the tension throughout your body beginning to flow away.

2. Clench your fists. Hold for seven to ten seconds and then release for fifteen to twenty seconds. Use these same intervals for all other muscle groups.

3. Tighten your biceps by drawing your forearms up toward your shoulders and making a muscle with both arms. Hold . . . and then relax.

4. Tighten your triceps, the muscles on the undersides of your upper arms, by extending your arms out straight and locking your elbows. Hold . . . and then relax.

5. Tense the muscles in your forehead by raising your eyebrows as far as you can. Hold . . . and then relax. Imagine your forehead muscles becoming smooth and limp as they relax.

6. Tense the muscles around your eyes by clenching your eyelids tightly shut. Hold . . . and then relax. Imagine sensations of deep relaxation spreading all around the area of your eyes.

7. Tighten your jaw by opening your mouth so widely that you stretch the muscles around the hinges of your jaw. Hold . . . and then relax. Let your lips part and allow your jaw to hang loose.

8. Tighten the muscles in the back of your neck by pulling your head way back, as if you were going to touch your head to your back (be gentle with this muscle group to avoid injury). Focus only on tensing the muscles in your neck. Hold . . . and then relax. Since this area is often especially tight, it's good to do this tense-relax cycle twice.

9. Take a few deep breaths and tune in to the weight of your head sinking into whatever surface it is resting on.

10. Tighten your shoulders by raising them up as if you were going to touch your ears. Hold . . . and then relax.

11. Tighten the muscles around your shoulder blades by pushing your shoulder blades back as if you were going to touch them together. Hold the tension in your shoulder blades . . . and then relax. Since this area is often especially tense, you might repeat this tense-relax sequence twice.

12. Tighten the muscles of your chest by taking in a deep breath. Hold for up to ten seconds . . . Tand then release slowly. Imagine any excess tension in your chest floating away with the exhalation.

13. Tighten your stomach muscles by sucking your stomach in. Hold . . . and then release. Imagine a wave of relaxation spreading through your abdomen.

14. Tighten your lower back by arching it up. (You can omit this exercise if you have lower back pain.) Hold . . . and then relax.

15. Tighten your buttocks by pulling them together. Hold . . . and then relax. Imagine the muscles in your hips loose and limp.

16. Squeeze the muscles in your thighs all the way down to your knees. You will probably have to tighten your hips along with your thighs, since the thigh muscles attach at the pelvis. Hold . . . and then relax. Feel your thigh muscles smoothing out and relaxing completely.

17. Tighten your calf muscles by pulling your toes toward you (flex carefully to avoid cramps). Hold . . . and then relax.

18. Tighten your feet by curling your toes downward. Hold . . . and then relax.

19. Mentally scan your body for any areas of residual tension. If a particular area remains tense, repeat one or two tense-relax cycles for that group of muscles.

20. Now imagine a wave of relaxation slowly spreading over your body, starting at your head and gradually penetrating every muscle group all the way down to your toes.

When you have completed the progressive muscle relaxation exercise, you should feel completely relaxed.

One of the things you might consider doing is recording this entire progression on an audiotape that you can listen to while you are doing your PMR exercises. That way you don't have to worry about memorizing the sequence and you can simply concentrate on relaxing.

Deep Breathing

Progressive muscle relaxation is an important component of any relaxation program. However, there are some other techniques that you should be aware of as well. One of these is deep abdominal breathing. You may have heard the phrase "take a breath and slow down." This is the very essence of deep breathing.

It turns out that one of the things that we often forget to do in our daily life is breathe. We tend to carry our tension in our chest and take very shallow breaths. You may have experienced this yourself. This habit is especially common when you experience anxiety. One very easy and important way to relax is to breathe deeply. When you breathe deeply, this actually helps more oxygen get to your brain, which can in turn help produce a relaxation response.

It is one thing to take a few deep breaths. It is another thing entirely to take the time out of your day to lie down and do some breathing exercises. Again, don't shortchange yourself by thinking you don't have the time to lie down and breathe. This is your recovery we are talking about here. Take the time and you will assuredly get results.

What follows is another exercise from *Coping with Anxiety* (Bourne and Garano 2003) that you should employ frequently in order to reduce your anxiety.

EXERCISE: ABDOMINAL BREATHING

1. Note the level of tension you're feeling. Then place one hand on your abdomen right beneath your rib cage.

2. Inhale slowly and deeply though your nose into the bottom of your lungs; in other words, send the air as low down as you can. If you're breathing from your abdomen, your hand should actually rise. Your chest should move only slightly while your abdomen expands.

3. When you've taken a full breath, pause for a moment and then exhale slowly through your nose or mouth, depending on your preference. Be sure to exhale fully. As you exhale, allow your whole body to just let go (you might visualize your arms and legs going loose and limp like a rag doll).

4. Do ten slow, full abdominal breaths. Try to keep your breathing smooth and regular without gulping in a big breath or letting your breath out all at once. It will help to slow down your breathing if you slowly count to four on the inhale and then slowly count to four on the exhale. Use this count to slow down your breathing for a few breaths, then let it go. Remember to pause briefly at the end of each inhalation.

5. After you've slowed down your breathing, count from twenty down to one, counting backward one number with each exhalation. The process should go like this: Slow inhale . . . Pause . . . Slow exhale (twenty) Slow inhale . . . Pause . . . Slow exhale (nineteen) Slow inhale . . . Pause . . . Slow exhale (eighteen) and so on down to one. If you start to feel light-headed while practicing abdominal breathing, stop for fifteen to twenty seconds and breathe in your normal way, then start again.

6. Extend the exercise if you wish by doing two or three sets of abdominal breaths, remembering to count backward from twenty to one for each set. Five full minutes of abdominal breathing will have a pronounced effect in reducing anxiety or early symptoms of panic. Some people prefer to count from one to twenty instead. Feel free to do this if you wish.

Visualization

The last relaxation technique I will be teaching you in this chapter is visualization. Visualization does not have an immediate physical component to it the way that progressive muscle relaxation and deep breathing do. Nonetheless, it is a very powerful technique to reduce your anxiety.

I am sure that you have visualized many things in your life. Have you ever caught yourself daydreaming and on coming "back to reality" you felt like you were almost really in the place you were thinking about? This is basically what visualization is. However, directed visualization takes your mind to a specific place in order to produce a specific response.

For example, sit down and just think about a beach for a minute. The cool salt air, the roar of the ocean, the sand beneath your feet. How do you feel? A little more relaxed than before, I'll bet. Visualization takes this to a whole new level. By visualizing a situation, your mind will respond as if it were really in that situation. This can be a very useful bit of information to know when you are coping with anxiety. If you are feeling tense, simply visualize being in a place where your tension would vanish. Make sure that you really focus on making the details rich.

What we will be practicing here is a set of guided visualizations. Guided visualization is a kind of semihypnosis. Below you will be provided with a couple of scripts that you can record on audiotapes and listen to while you practice the visualizations. While listening to the tapes, really try to visualize as completely as you can all of the details that are being spoken to you. You will want to be as relaxed as possible when you do the visualizations, so follow the same principles that you did when preparing for the progressive muscle relaxation exercises: find a quiet spot where you won't be interrupted, get comfortable, and let your worry drop away. You will be able to visualize much better when you are in a relaxed state. I would suggest doing some abdominal breathing or even a cycle of PMR before starting your visualization exercise.

EXERCISE: GUIDED VISUALIZATION

What follows are two different scripts from *Coping with Anxiety* (Bourne and Garano 2003) that you will want to record on audiotapes and then listen to and visualize with when you are prepared to start a guided visualization. You can also buy a guided visualization tape of your choice.

Walking on a Beach

You're walking down a long wooden stairway to a beautiful, expansive beach. It looks almost deserted and stretches off into the distance as far as you can see. The sand is very fine and light . . . almost white in appearance. You step onto the sand in your bare feet and rub it between your toes. It feels so good to walk slowly along this beautiful beach. The roaring sound of the surf is so soothing that you can just let go of anything on your mind. You're watching the waves ebb and flow . . . they are slowly coming in . . . breaking over each other . . . and then slowly flowing back out again. The ocean itself is a very beautiful shade of blue . . . a shade of blue that is so relaxing just to look at. You look out over the surface of the ocean all the way to the horizon, and then follow the horizon as far as you can see, noticing how it bends slightly downward as it follows the curvature of the earth. As you scan the ocean you can see, many miles offshore, a tiny sailboat skimming along the surface of the water. And all these sights help you to just let go and relax even more. As you continue walking down the beach, you become aware of the fresh, salty smell of the sea air. You take in a deep breath . . . breathe out . . . and feel very refreshed and even more relaxed. Overhead you notice two seagulls flying out to sea . . . looking very graceful as they soar into the wind . . . and you imagine how you might feel yourself if you had the freedom to fly. You find yourself settling into a deep state of relaxation as you continue walking down the beach. You feel the sea breeze blowing gently against your cheek and the warmth of the sun overhead penetrating your neck and shoulders. The warm, liquid sensation of the sun just relaxes you even more . . . and you're beginning to feel perfectly content on this beautiful beach. It's such a lovely day. In a moment, up ahead, you see a comfortable-looking beach chair. Slowly, you begin to approach the beach chair . . . and when you finally reach it, you sit back and settle in. Lying back in this comfortable beach chair, you let go and relax even more, drifting even deeper into relaxation. In a little while you might close your eyes and just listen to the sound of the surf, the unending cycle of waves ebbing and flowing. And the rhythmic sound of the surf carries you even deeper . . . deeper still . . . into a wonderful state of quietness and peace.

Walking in the Forest

You're walking along a path deep in the forest. All around you there are tall trees . . . pine, fir, redwood, oak . . . try to see them. The rushing sound of the wind blowing through the treetops is so soothing, allowing you to let go. You can smell the rich dampness of the forest floor, the smell of earth, and new seedlings, and rotting leaves. Now you look up through the treetops until you can see a light blue sky. You notice how high the sun is in the sky. As the sun enters the canopy of the treetops, it splinters into rays that penetrate through the trees to the forest floor. You're watching the intricate patterns of light and dark created as the light filters down through the trees. The forest feels like a great primeval cathedral . . . filling you with a sense of peace and reverence for all living things. Off in the distance, you can hear the sound of rushing water echoing through the forest. It gets louder as you approach, and before long you are at the edge of a mountain stream. You're looking at the stream, noticing how clear and sparkling the water is. Imagine sitting down and making yourself very comfortable. You might sit down on a flat rock up against a tree or you might even decide to lie down on a grassy slope. You can see the mountain stream creating rapids as it moves, rushing around a variety of large and small rocks. These rocks are many shades of brown, gray, and white and some are covered with moss. You can see the sparkling water rushing over some and around others, making whirlpools and eddies. The rushing sound of the water is so peaceful that you can just let yourself drift . . . relaxing more and more. You take in a deep breath of fresh air and breathe out, finding the subtle smells of the forest very refreshing. As you let yourself sink into the soft bed of grass or dead leaves or fragrant pine needles beneath you, let go of any strains or concerns . . . allowing the sights, sounds, and smells of this beautiful forest to fill you with a deep sense of peace.

Coming Out of a Visualization

When you have completed your visualization exercise, bring yourself back to a fully awake and aware state of mind with the following statement (you can record this at the end of your visualization tape):

Now in a moment you can come back to an alert, wakeful state of mind. Pay attention as I count from one up to five. When I get up to five, you can open your eyes and feel awake, alert, and refreshed. One . . . gradually beginning to come back to an alert, wakeful state of mind. Two . . .

more and more awake. Three . . . beginning to move your hands and feet as you become more alert. Four . . . almost back to a fully alert state. And five . . . opening your eyes now, finding yourself fully awake, alert, and refreshed.

Remember that this kind of relaxation is a form of semi-hypnosis. It is very relaxing and perfectly safe, but you need to make sure to take some precautions. When you are finished, you should get up slowly and walk around for a little while to get yourself grounded again. It is also important that you refrain from driving a motor vehicle or doing any strenuous activity for at least ten minutes after you have completed the exercise.

RELAXATION EVERY DAY

You now have at your disposal some of the most powerful techniques to combat anxiety that psychology has to offer. As I said earlier in the chapter, in order to make the most out of these exercises you really need to incorporate them into your daily life. Try to create and keep a regular relaxation schedule. It may sound silly, but doing this stuff every day will make a huge difference in your life.

I would also like to point out here that while these strategies are incredibly powerful, if you are experiencing ongoing problems with anxiety, you should seek professional help. As with depression, anxiety is a very serious psychological issue. If you feel that your anxiety is more than you can handle alone, see a therapist. All of the same advice applies to seeking professional help for anxiety as it does for depression. Part of learning how to help yourself is learning when to know you need help.

There are also several excellent books on the market for anxiety issues. Two are *Coping with Anxiety* (which many of the exercises in this chapter are borrowed from—thank you, Dr. Bourne) and *The Anxiety and Phobia Workbook*, both available from New Harbinger Publications.

Putting It All Together

Congratulations! You have now finished *The Mild Traumatic Brain Injury Workbook* and you should be well on the road to recovery.

Before putting the book down, it's time to do a final review of the goals that you set in chapter 5. I believe that this will help you to see not only how far you have come, but where you still need to go.

GOALS REVIEW

Earlier in the book, you listed the symptoms that you were suffering from most, and you then developed these symptoms into a list of goals. Let's complete this goal exercise with a review.

EXERCISE: GOALS REVIEW

Part I: Initial Goals. Please list your initial goals here:

1. _____

2. _____

3. _____

4. _____

5. _____

Part II: Restated Goals. Please list your goals as you restated them in chapter 5 here:

1. _____

2. _____

3. _____

4. _____

5. _____

Part III: How Well Did You Do?

Now I would like you to rank each of your goals on a simple rating scale. In the table below, please circle the number that best applies to how well you feel you did in accomplishing each of the five goals you listed above. A ranking of 1 means you did not do as well as you expected to, a ranking of 2 means that you did about as well as you expected to, and a ranking of 3 means that you did better than you expected to.

Please rate your goals now. (If you chose to list more goals on your own, it would be helpful for you to rank these as well.)

	Less than expected	As expected	Better than expected
Goal 1	1	2	3
Goal 2	1	2	3
Goal 3	1	2	3
Goal 4	1	2	3
Goal 5	1	2	3

Now you can make an assessment about your own achievements through this book. If you did better than you expected, or about as well as you expected, give yourself a pat on the back. Your hard work is paying off, and you are recovering. If you did not do quite as well as you expected, don't get discouraged. Remember that recovery is a long process. Rest assured, you will get better. I have seen many patients in my years of treating people who have suffered MTBI, and there is always some improvement over time.

Areas You Still Want to Work On

If you did not do as well as you expected, or if there are some areas that you would like to improve upon, please go back to those particular sections in the book and review them. Though you have already completed all of the puzzles, you can use the exercises in each chapter as a model. There are many puzzle books on the market that have exercises very similar to many of the exercises in this book. Help yourself recover by going to the store to pick up a few of these books.

There are also a lot of books, self-help and otherwise, about different areas covered in this book. You will be exercising your mind by simply doing the research to find these types of books. Take a trip to your local library and see what you can find. Or go to a bookstore and see what they have in the health and psychology sections that appeals to you.

There is a resources section at the back of this book as well. This is presented to help you further your recovery. Contact information and Web sites are provided. There are many people out there who are available to help you further your recovery. Take advantage of what they have to offer.

IN CLOSING

Now we are at the end. I would like to say that it has been a pleasure writing this book for you. I truly hope that the information and exercises in the book have helped you on your road to recovery. Keep up the hard work, and you will get better.

Before we close, I would like to leave you with this inspirational story.

The Meaning of Life

Minister Phillips stood before his congregation with several items in front of him. As the church quieted down, he quietly picked up a large, empty jar and proceeded to fill it with rocks. He then looked up into the church crowd and asked, "Is the jar full?" The congregation agreed that it was.

Minister Phillips then quietly picked up a handful of pebbles and poured them into the jar. He shook the jar lightly, which allowed the pebbles to roll into the open areas between the rocks. He then asked the congregation again whether the jar was full. Unanimously, they agreed it was.

The minister then picked up a bag of sand and poured it into the jar. The sand filled the spaces between the pebbles. "Now is the jar full?" asked Minister Phillips. "Yes!" the congregation immediately replied.

"Now," said the minister, as the laughter subsided, "I want you to recognize that this jar represents your life. The rocks are the important things—your family, your children, your spouse, your health—

things that if everything else was lost and only they remained, your life would still be full. The pebbles are the other things that matter like your career, money, your house and car. The sand is everything else—the small stuff.

"If you put the sand into the jar first, there is no room for the pebbles or the rocks. The same goes for your life. If you spend all your time and energy on the small stuff, you will never have room for the things that are important to you. Pay attention to the things that are critical to your happiness. Play with your children, listen to your partner, take care of your health.

"Take vacations, enjoy your family and friends, and take your partner out dancing. There will always be time to clean the house, work late, or fix the car. Take care of the rocks first because they really matter. Set your priorities, and the rocks will take care of the pebbles. The rest is just sand." With a long, reflective pause Minister Phillips looked into the crowd. "Now go on your way and don't worry about the sand."

APPENDIX A

Glossary/Pronunciation and Comprehension Answer Key

Amygdala: Almond shaped nucleus in the temporal lobe that plays a role in memory and emotional control.

Angular gyrus: Located in the temporal-parietal-occipital area; involved with processing sensory information.

Anterior: Pertaining to the front part of a structure.

Aphasia/dysphasia: Inability to use language to communicate and/or comprehend due to brain cell damage; impairment in speech. Dysphasia is a milder form of aphasia. *Receptive aphasia* is impairment in the comprehension of speech. *Expressive aphasia* is difficulty in verbally expressing oneself.

Arcuate fasciculus: Fibers connecting the superior and middle frontal convolutions with the temporal lobe and temporal pole.

Association: Your mind stores memory in a series of associations that are tied together in a logical manner. Association serves as a trigger that stimulates the retrieval of the specific memory needed. Association can be used as a tool in both recall and encoding.

Auditory association area: Portion of the cortex that processes auditory information.

Auditory cortex: Portion of the cortex that processes auditory information.

Brain stem: The rear lower part of the brain, just above the spinal cord. It contains the midbrain, the pons, and the medulla oblongata, structures that control breathing and heartbeat, and serves as a relay station for all motion and sensation.

Broca's area: Area of the brain controlling speech, located in the lower part of the left frontal lobe.

Cerebellum: The portion of the brain that is located below the cerebrum and is concerned with coordinating movements.

Cingulate gyrus: An arch shpaed gyrus lying above the corpus callosum that communicates information between the two hemispheres of the brain.

Comprehension: The ability to understand things that are heard, seen, and/or touched.

Cortical: Relating to the cortex, the outer layer of the brain.

Cranial auditory nerves: Number eight of twelve paired nerves, these assist in hearing.

Elaboration: The level of processing involved with learning information.

Extrapyramidal system: Part of the central nervous system; coordinates body movements.

Fornix: Bands of white fibers in each cerebral hemisphere.

Frontal lobe: The area of the brain located at the front, closest to the forehead. It is responsible for emotions, behaviors, social and motor skills, abstract thinking, reasoning, planning, judgment, and memory.

Frontal association cortex: In movement, the primary motor areas receive information from the premotor areas and the premotor areas receive information from the frontal premotor association cortex.

Frontal premotor association cortex: Integrates sensory and motor functions.

Hemisphere: Outer regions of the brain that make up higher order functioning. There are two hemipsheres in the brain, the left and the right.

Hypothalamus: The part of the brain that influences sex drive, sleep, body temperature, appetite, long-term memory, and the expression of emotion.

Lateral: Occurring on one side of the body.

Limbic system: A group of interconnected deep-brain structures that helps the hypothalamus prioritize incoming information and also plays a part in controlling memory and emotion.

Mammillary bodies: Located in the hypothalamus; associated with memory and retrieval functions.

Mammillothalamic tract: Located in front of the thalamus; involved in memory and emotions.

Motor strip: Part of the cortical brain that is devoted to processing motor movements.

Neural impulses: A signal moving along the nerve.

Occipital lobe: The posterior, or back, part of the brain. This area is involved in perceiving and understanding visual information.

Olfactory: Pertaining to the sense of smell.

Parahippocampal gyrus: Located in the most medial basal part of the temporal lobe; integrates sensory information with data from within the brain.

Parietal lobe: The upper middle section of the brain. This area is responsible for sensory and spatial awareness, giving feedback from and understanding of eye, hand, and arm movements during complex operations such as reading, writing, and numerical calculations.

Perception: Ability to accurately interpret internal and external sensory information.

Postcentral gyrus: Located behind the central fissure; causes sensation to the skin surface.

Posterior: Pertaining to the back part of the brain.

Premotor frontal cortex: Includes premotor, frontal eye fields, and Broca's area.

Primary visual cortex: Part of the neocortex that receives visual input from the retina.

Pyramidal system: Begins in the cerebellum; regulates and coordinates muscle movement.

Sensorimotor cortex: Area of the brain that controls movement and sensation.

Sensory strip: Located in cerebrum; controls the five senses.

Somesthetic sensations: Pain, temperature, and nondiscriminative touch.

Subcortical: Part of the brain below the cerebral cortex.

Subcortical gray matter: The gray matter regions are the areas where the actual processing is done, whereas the white matter provides the communication between different gray matter areas and between the gray matter and the rest of the body.

Superior longitudinal fasciculus: Fiber bundle connecting the frontal lobe center to the parietal, occipital, and temporal lobes.

Superior temporal gyrus: Houses the auditory cortex; area receiving and processing auditory sensations.

Supplementary motor cortex: The area next to the pirmary motor cortex involved in the initiation of voluntary movements.

Supramarginal gyrus: A small area of the parietal lobe important in the selection and combining of word meanings with word forms.

Sylvian fissure: The dividing line between the temporal, parietal, and frontal lobes.

Temporal lobe: A part of the brain located beneath the frontal and parietal lobes that plays a part in remembering information, noticing things, understanding music, categorizing objects, the ability to smell and taste, and sexual and aggressive behavior. At the back of the left temporal lobe is Wernicke's area, which is responsible for hearing and interpreting language.

Thalamus: Part of the brain that acts as a nerve-impulse relay station for information being sent to and from the brain, passing it to the hypothalamus to be screened and transmitted throughout the body.

Uncus: Anterior part of parahippocampal gyrus; hook shaped.

Vestibular system: Senses movement of the head; located in the middle ear.

Visual association cortex: Integrates data from the primary visual cortex to create orientation, movement, color, three dimensions, and spatial location of things.

Wernicke's area: An area of the brain that is involved with processing language.

APPENDIX B

Resources

ABLEDATA System: (800) 227-0216, www.abledata.com. Information on assistive technology.

ADA Information Line: (202) 514-0301

Agency for Health Care Administration: (800) 342-0828. Publishes information on nursing homes.

AGS Foundation for Health and Aging: (212) 755-6810, www.healthinaging.org

Alternative Medicine Connection: www.arxc.com

American Academy of Neurology: (612) 695-2791, (800) 879-1960, www.aan.com

American Academy of Ophthalmology: (415) 561-8500, www.aao.org

American Academy of Otolaryngology—Head and Neck Surgery: (703) 836-4444, www.entnet.org

American Academy of Physical Medicine and Rehabilitation: (800) 825-6582, www.aapmr.org

American Association of Electrodiagnostic Medicine: (507) 288-0100, www.aaem.net

American Association of Neuroscience Nurses: (888) 557-2266, www.aann.org

American Association of Oriental Medicine: (610) 266-1433, www.aaom.org

American Association of Sex Educators, Counselors, and Therapists: (319) 895-8407

American Chiropractic Association: (703) 276-8800, www.amerchiro.org

American Chronic Pain Association: (916) 632-0922, www.theacpa.org

American College of Emergency Physicians: (800) 798-1822, www.acep.org

American Council for Headache Education: (800) 255-ACHE, www.achenet.org

American Dance Therapy Association: (410) 997-4040, www.adta.org

American Epilepsy Society: (860) 586-7505, www.aesnet.org

American Headache Society: (856) 423-0043, www.ahsnet.org

American Hearing Research Foundation: (312) 726-9670, www.american-hearing.org

American Massage Therapy Association: (847) 864-0123

American Medical Association: (312) 464-5000, www.ama-assn.org

American Neurological Association: (612) 545-6284, www.aneuroa.org

American Occupational Therapy Association: (301) 652-2682

American Osteopathic Association: (800) 621-1773, www.osteopathic.org

American Pain Society: (847) 375-4715, www.ampainsoc.org

American Physical Therapy Association: (800) 999-2782, www.apta.org

American Polarity Therapy Association: (303) 545-2080, www.polaritytherapy.org

American Psychiatric Association: (202) 682-6000, www.psych.org

American Psychological Association: (202) 336-5500, www.apa.org

American Society of Clinical Hypnosis: (847) 297-3317, www.asch.net

American Society of Neuroimaging: (612) 545-6291, www.asnweb.org

American Society of Neurorehabilitation: (612) 545-6324, www.asnr.com

American Speech-Language-Hearing Association: (800) 498-2071, www.asha.org

American Tinnitus Association: (503) 248-9985, www.ata.org

Association for Applied Psychophysiology and Biofeedback: (303) 422-8436, www.aapb.org

Association for Research in Vision and Ophthalmology: (301) 571-1844, www.arvo.org

Association of University Professors of Neurology: (612) 545-6724, www.aupn.org

Better Hearing Institute: (703) 642-0580, www.betterhearing.org

Biofeedback Certification Institute of America: (303) 420-2902

Brain Injury Association of America: (800) 444-6443, www.biausa.org

California Yoga Teachers' Association: (800) 395-8075

Center for Assistive Technology: (816) 931-2121

Center for Coping: (516) 822-3131

Centre for Neuro Skills: TBI Resource Guide, www.neuroskills.com

Child Neurology Society: (651) 486-9447, www.childneurologysociety.org

Citizens United for Research in Epilepsy: (630) 734-9957, www.cureepilepsy.org

Commission for Accreditation of Rehabilitation Facilities: (520) 325-1044, www.carf.org

Crestwood Company: (414) 352-5678, www.communicationaids.com

Depression Awareness, Recognition, and Treatment: (800) 421-4211

Dystonia Medical Research Foundation: (800) 377-3978, www.dystonia-foundation.org

Easter Seal Society: (800) 221-6827, www.easterseals.com. Consult your local phone directory for your local office.

Epilepsy Foundation of America: (800) 332-1000, www.epilepsyfoundation.org.

Epilepsy Services of Southeast Florida: (561) 478-6515

Evelyn Wood Reading Dynamics: (800) 447-7323

Feldenkrais Guild: (541) 926-0981, www.feldenkrais.com

Grief Recovery Hotline: (800) 445-4808

Herb Research Foundation: (303) 449-2265, www.herbs.org

Homeopathic Educational Services: (510) 649-0294, www.homeopathic.com

Hospice: Consult your local directory for your local office; National Hospice (800) 658-8898.

House Ear Institute: (213) 483-4431, www.hei.org

Insurance Information Institute: (800) 331-9146, www.iii.org

Internet Mental Health Home Page: www.mentalhealth.com

Kenneth I. Kolpan, Esq.: (617) 426-2558. Brain injury lawyer.

The Learning Company: (800) 227-5609, www.learningco.com

Learning Disabilities Association of America: (412) 341-1515, www.ldanatl.org

MedicineNet: www.medicinenet.com

Meniere's Network Ear Foundation: (615) 329-7807, www.earfoundation.com

Movement Disorder Society: (414) 276-2145, www.movementdisorders.org

Muscular Dystrophy Association: (602) 529-2000, (800) 572-1717, www.mdausa.org

National Association of State Head Injury Administrators: (301) 656-3500, www.nashia.org

National Center for Homeopathy: (703) 548-7790, www.homeopathic.org

National Center for Learning Disabilities: (212) 545-7510, www.ncld.org

National Center for Victims of Crime: (703) 276-2880, www.nvc.org

National Chronic Care Consortium: (952) 814-2652, www.nccconline.org

National Commission for the Certification of Acupuncturists: (202) 232-1404

National Consumers League: (202) 835-3323

National Council on Aging: (800) 424-9046

National Eye Institute: (301) 496-5248, www.nei.nih.gov

National Eye Research Foundation: (847) 564-4652, www.nerf.org

National Family Caregivers Association: (800) 896-3650, www.nfcacares.org

National Headache Foundation: (888) 643-5552, www.headaches.org

National Institute of Deafness and Other Communication Disorders: (800) 241-1055, www.nidcd .nih.gov

National Institute of Neurological Disorders and Stroke: (800) 352-9424, www.ninds.nih.gov

National Institutes of Health: (301) 496-4000, www.nih.gov

National Insurance Consumer Hotline: (800) 942-4242

National Organization for Rare Disorders: (800) 999-6673, www.rarediseases.org

National Organization for Victim Assistance: (202) 232-6682, www.try-nova.org

National Rehabilitation Information Center: (800) 346-2742, www.naric.com

The Neurotrauma Law Nexus: www.neurolaw.com

Nightingale-Conant: (800) 323-5552, www.nightingale.com. Books and audio products for personal growth.

Northeast Rehabilitation Health Networ: (603) 893-2900, www.northeastrehab.com

The Orton Dyslexia Society: (800) 222-3123, www.selu.edu/Academics/Education/TEC/orton.htm

Outdoor Camping, Camp Hemlocks, Massachusetts Brain Association: (800) 242-0030. Camp for adults with TBI designed to promote independence and summer fun.

The People's Pharmacy: P.O. Box 52027, Durham, NC 27717, mail only. Dispenses info about medication.

The Perspectives Network: (334) 639-5037, (800) 685-6302, www.tbi.org

Pulse Data HumanWare: (800) 772-3393, www.pulsedata.com. Products and solutions for people with visual impairments.

Recovery of Male Potency: (810) 357-1314

Respite Care: Provides assistance with health care; consult your local phone directory

Social Security Administration—Medicare and Medicaid: (800) 772-1213.

Society for Clinical and Experimental Hypnosis: (317) 228-8073, http://ijceh.educ.wsu.edu/sceh/scehframe.htm

Society for Neuroscience: (202) 462-6688, www.sfn.org

Speak Easy International Foundation: (201) 262-0895

Sportime International: (800) 444-5700, www.sportime.com. Offers specialized rehabilitative equipment for fun and movement.

Stoler, Diane Roberts, Ed.D.: (978) 352-6349. Makes contacts with other brain-injured people.

Taste and Smell Center, University of Connecticut Health Center: (800) 679-2000

United Parkinson Foundation: (312) 733-1893

United Way: Consult your local phone directory

University of Pittsburgh Alternative Medicine Home Page: www.pitt.edu/~cbw/altm.html

U.S. Department of Health and Human Services: (800) 358-9295

U.S. Department of Labor Office of Disability Employment Policy: (866) 633-7365, www.dol.gov/odep

Vestibular Disorders Association: (503) 229-7705, www.vestibular.com

Visiting Nurse Association: www.vnaa.org. Provides medical assistance; consult your local phone directory.

Widowed Persons Service: (800) 424-3410

Xerox Imaging System: (800) 248-6550, www.xerox.com

Yahoo-Health Directory on Neurology: www.yahoo.com/health/medicine/neurology

APPENDIX C

Answers to Exercises and Puzzles

CHAPTER 1

EXERCISE: LETTER SEARCH ANSWERS

Check your answers for the timed Letter Search below.

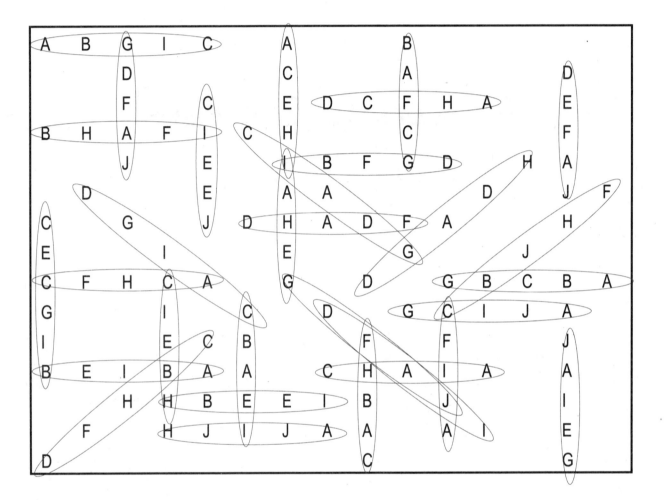

ABGIC	JAFDG	DHADF	IAHEG	IEEBH	CFIJA
DCFHA	CFHCA	CBJHF	DFAJI	DEFAJ	CIEBH
CIADG	GEIAJ	AJIJH	IEABC	CAIGD	DGFBI
BAFCG	ABIEB	CABHF	DFHBC	ABCBG	ACEHI
BHAFI	DGADH	CIEEJ	CHAIA	CECGI	GCIJA

CHAPTER 2

EXERCISE: MAZE 1 ANSWER

Compare your solution to Maze 1 with the one provided below.

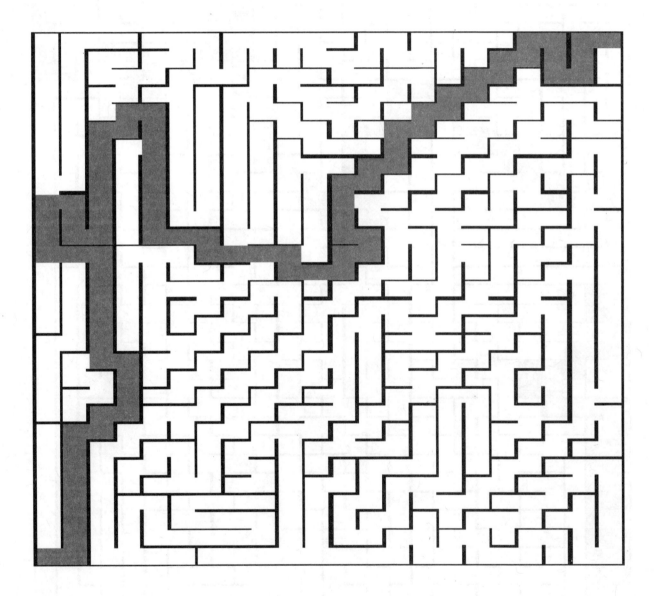

CHAPTER 3

EXERCISE: MAZE 2 ANSWER

Compare your solution to Maze 2 with the one provided below.

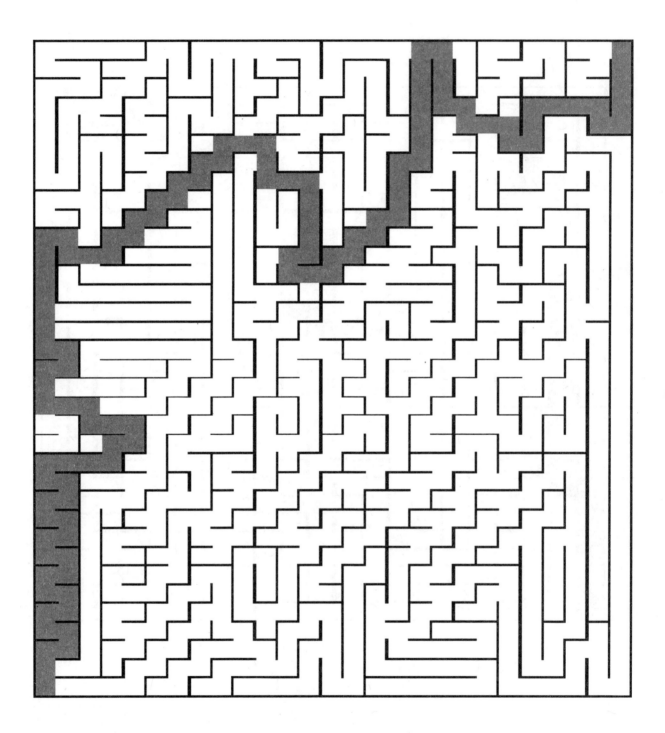

CHAPTER 4

EXERCISE: COGNITIVE ANAGRAMS ANSWERS

1.	Selves	Vessel
2.	BIT	TBI
3.	Scorbutical	Subcortical
4.	ACT	CAT
5.	RIM	MRI
6.	Brumal	Lumbar
7.	Snipe	Spine
8.	Nesses	Senses
9.	Daimon	Domain
10	.Renal	Learn

EXERCISE: MAZE 3 ANSWER

Compare your solution to Maze 3 Exercise with the one provided below.

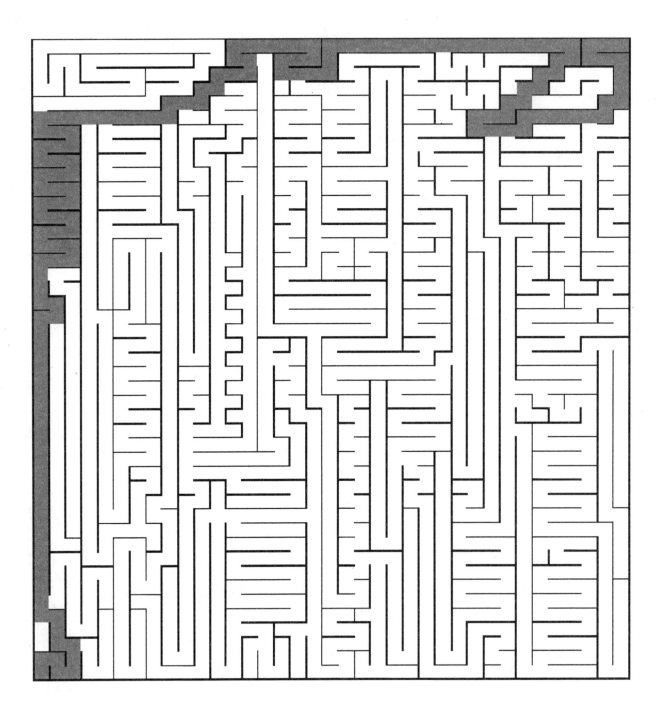

CHAPTER 5

EXERCISE: MAZE 4 ANSWERS

Compare your solution to Maze 4 with the one provided below.

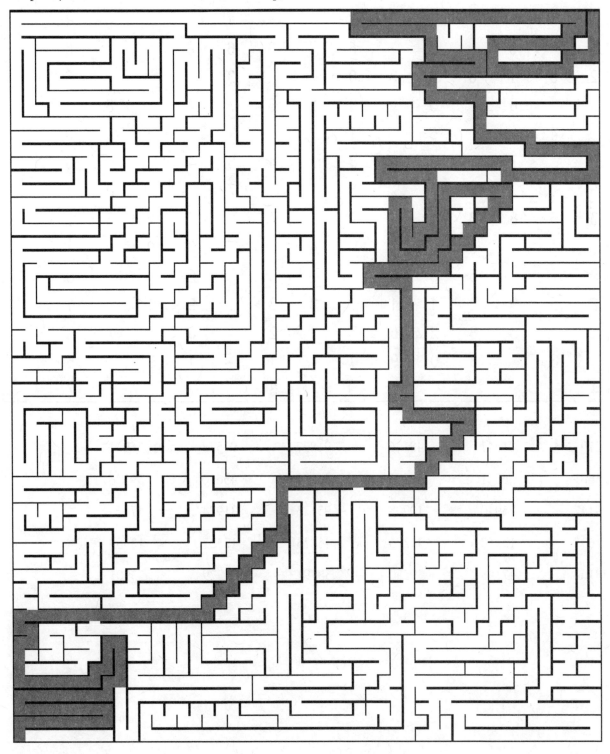

EXERCISE: NUMBER SEARCH ANSWERS

Check your answers for the timed Number Search below.

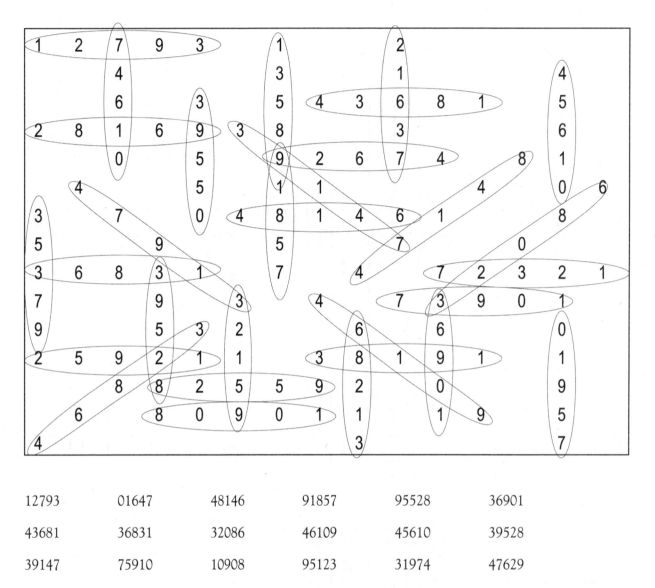

12793	01647	48146	91857	95528	36901
43681	36831	32086	46109	45610	39528
39147	75910	10908	95123	31974	47629
21637	12952	31286	46823	12327	13589
28169	47148	39550	38191	35379	73901

CHAPTER 6

Compare your solution to Maze 5 with the one provided below.

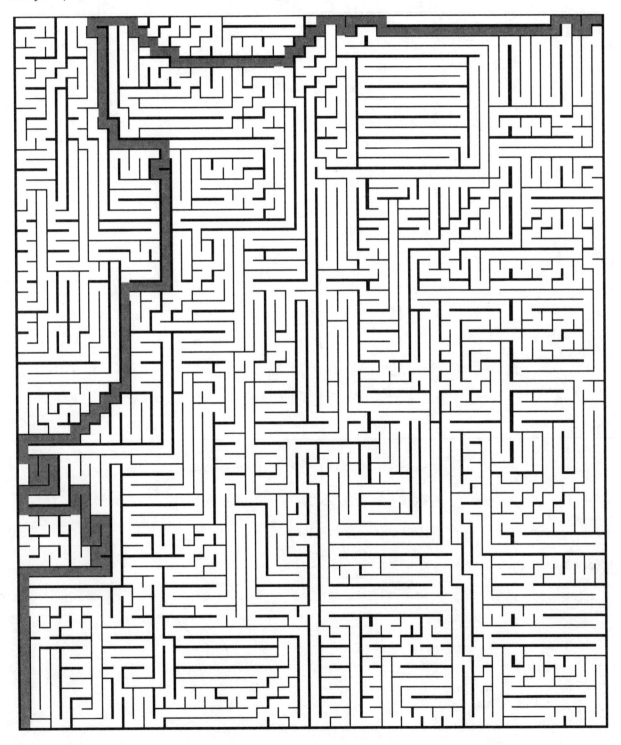

CHAPTER 7

EXERCISE: SYMBOL SEARCH ANSWERS

Check your answers for the timed Symbol Search below.

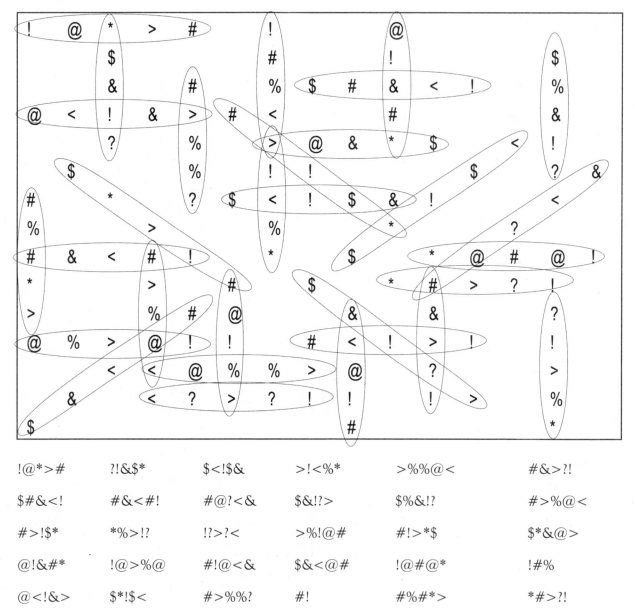

!@*>#	?!&$*	$<!$&	>!<%*	>%%@<	#&>?!
$#&<!	#&<#!	#@?<&	$&!?>	$%&!?	#>%@<
#>!$*	*%>!?	!?>?<	>%!@#	#!>*$	$*&@>
@!&#*	!@>%@	#!@<&	$&<@#	!@#@*	!#%
@<!&>	$*!$<	#>%%?	#!	#%#*>	*#>?!

CHAPTER 8

Compare your solution to Maze 6 with the one provided below.

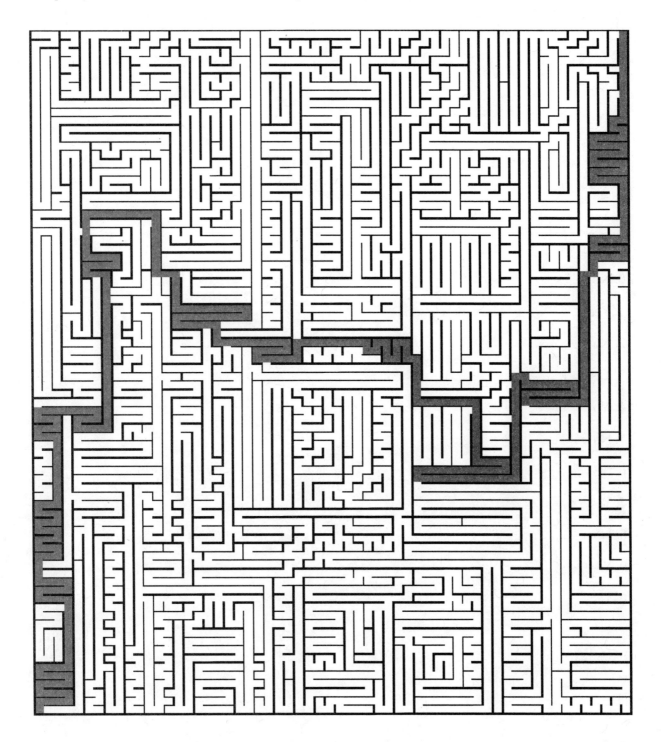

CHAPTER 10

EXERCISE: ATTIC CLEANING ANSWERS

1. Yes

2. No

3. Yes

4. No

5. Yes

6. No

7. Yes

8. Yes

9. No

10. No

11. Yes

12. No

13. Yes

14. No

15. No

16. No

17. Yes

18. No

19. Yes

20. Yes

CHAPTER 11

1. Ballpoint is part of a   pen

2. Steering wheel is part of a   car

3. Pedal is part of a   bicycle

4. Foot is part of the   leg

5. Knob is part of a   door

6. Page is part of a   book

7. Bulb is part of a   light

8. Limb is part of a   tree

9. Speaker is part of a   stereo

10. Collar is part of a   shirt

11. Blade is part of a   knife

12. Leaf is part of a   tree

13. Tile is part of a   floor

14. Lace is part of a   shoe

15. A pip is part of a   fruit

16. A filament is part of a   light bulb

17. Decimal is part of a   number

18. An oar is part of a   boat

19. Iris is part of an   eye

20. Cuticle is part of the   fingernail

21. Incus (anvil) is part of the   ear

22. Hippocampus is part of the   brain

23. Heel is part of the   foot

24. Bark is part of a   tree

25. A wick is part of a   candle

26. Aileron is part of an   airplane's wing or wing

27. Cones and rods are parts of an   eye

28. An inning is part of a   baseball game

29. A stirrup is part of a   saddle

30. A ripcord is part of a   parachute

31. A bride is part of a   wedding or marriage

32. Type is part of a   printing press

33. A pimento is part of an   olive

34. A bayonet is part of a   rifle

35. An inauguration is part of a   presidency

36. RAM is part of a   computer

37. A piston is part of an   engine

38. A mouse is part of a   computer

39. A cavity is part of a   tooth

40. A margin is part of a   page

41. A talon is part of a   bird's foot

42. A lash is part of an   eye

43. A pillar is part of a   building

44. A shingle is part of a   roof

45. A treble clef is part of   music

46. A scalpel is part of a   surgery kit

47. Corolla is part of a   flower

48. A cob is part of an   ear of corn

49. A noun is part of a   sentence

50. A radiator is part of a   car

EXERCISE: WORD PUZZLES ANSWERS

Below are the answers to the word puzzles.

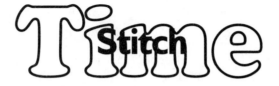

Answer: A stitch in time

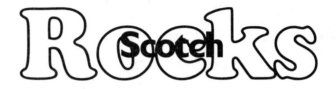

Answer: Scotch on the rocks

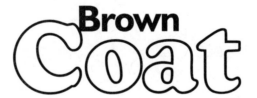

Answer: Brown overcoat

ATTE(N)TION

Answer: Center of attention

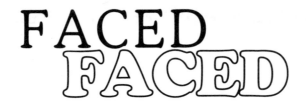

FACED
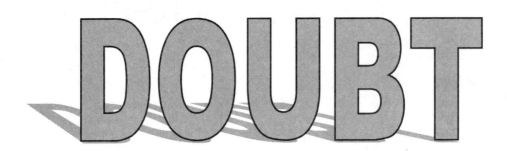

Answer: Two-faced

Answer: Shadow of a doubt

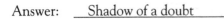

MID caught DLE

Answer: Caught in the middle

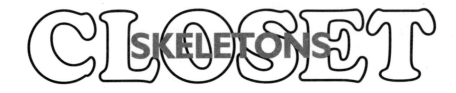

Answer: Skeletons in the closet

CHAPTER 12

Below are the answers to the Block Decipher exercise.

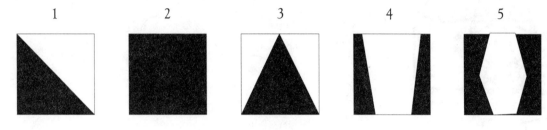

3	1	2	1
5	2	1	4
4	3	1	5
3	1	1	4

EXERCISE: VISUAL DISCRIMINATION ANSWER

The X indicates the correct answer.

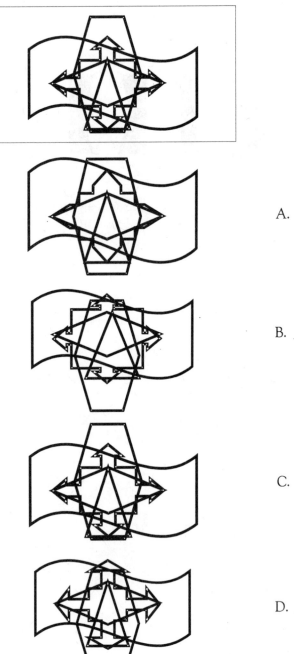

A. _____

B. _____

C. __X____

D. _____

EXERCISE: LOCATE THE REGIONS OF THE BRAIN

See the answers on the brain drawing below.

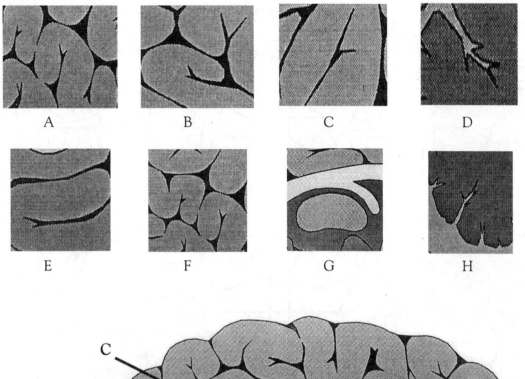

A   B   C   D

E   F   G   H

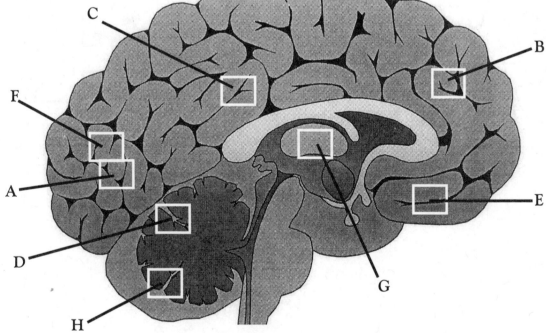

EXERCISE: FIGURE GROUND ANSWERS

Below are the answers to the Figure Ground exercise. The correct figures are shaded.

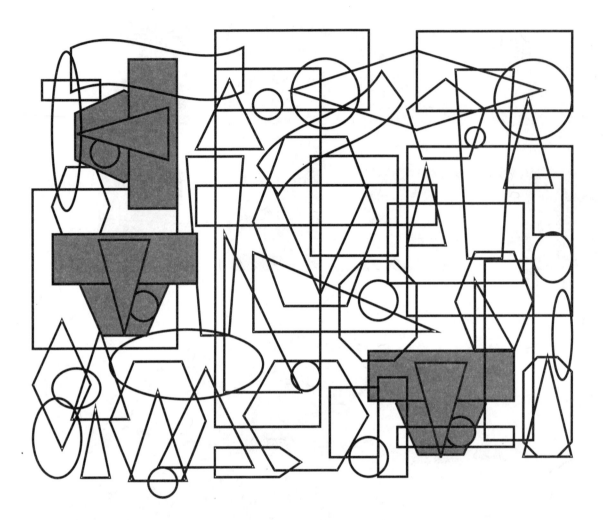

References

American Psychiatric Association. 1994. *Quick Reference to the Diagnostic Criteria from the Diagnostic and Statistical Manual of Mental Disorders.* 4th ed. Washington DC: American Psychiatric Association.

American Speech-Language-Hearing Association. 2004a. Roles of speech-language pathologists in the identification, diagnosis, and treatment of individuals with cognitive-communication disorders. Position statement. *ASHA Supplement,* 24, in press.

American Speech-Language-Hearing Association. 1983. *Committee on Language: Definition of Language.* ASHA 25(6), 44.

Atkinson, R. C., and R. M. Shiffrin. 1968. Human memory: A proposed system and its control processes. In *The Psychology of Learning and Motivation,* vol. 2, edited by K. W. Spence and J. T. Spence. Orlando, Fla.: Academic Press.

Bourne, E., and L. Garano. 2003. *Coping with Anxiety.* Oakland, Calif.: New Harbinger Publications.

Brink, T. L., J. A. Yesavage, O. Lum, P. Heersema, M. B. Adey, and T. L. Rose. 1982. Screening tests for geriatric depression. *Clinical Gerontologist* 1:37-44.

Centers for Disease Control and Prevention. 2003. *Program in Brief: Monitoring Traumatic Injury in the United States: An Interim Report to Congress.* Atlanta, Ga.: Centers for Disease Control and Prevention. M. C. Mann, P. Patterson, and M Helfand.

Chestnut, R. M., N. Carney, and H. Maynard. 1999. Summary report and evidence for the effectiveness of rehabilitation for persons with traumatic brain injury. *Journal of Head Trauma Rehabilitation* 148:176-188.

Cohen, A. 2003. About Vision and Brain Injuries. From www.braininjuries.org. Downloaded August 11, 2003.

Goodwin, D. W., B. Powell, D. Bremer, H. Hoine, and J. Stern. 1969. Alcohol and recall: State dependent effects in man. *Science* 163:1358.

Hamby, J. 2000. Vision and Perception: The adult patient with brain injury or stroke. Seminar presented in Pompano Beach, Fla..

Helm-Estabrooks, N., and M. Albert. 1991. *Manual of Aphasia Therapy*. Austin, Tex.: Pro-Ed.

Horn, L., and N. Zasler (eds.). 1992. Neuromedical diagnosis and management of post-concussive disorders in rehabilitation of post-concussive disorders. *Physical Medicine and Rehabilitation State of the Art Reviews*. Philadelphia: Hanley and Belfus, Inc.

Jennett, B., and G. Teasdale. 1981. *Management of Head Injuries*. Philadelphia: F. A. Davis.

Lezak, M. D. 1995. *Neuropsychological Assessment*. 3rd ed. New York: Oxford University Press.

National Association of State Head Injury Administrators. 2001. Traumatic brain injury facts: Emergency medical services. Fact sheet available from NASHIA, 4733 Bethesda Ave., Suite 330, Bethesda, MD 20816, www.nashia.org.

Parente, R., and M. Stapleton. 1993. An empowerment model of memory training. *Applied Cognitive Psychology* 7:585-602.

Paterson, R. 2002. *Your Depression Map*. Oakland, Calif.: New Harbinger Publications.

Sheikh, J. I., J. A. Yesavage, J. O. Brooks, L. F. Friedman, P. Gratzinger, R. D. Hill, A. Zadeik, and T. Crook. 1991. Proposed factor structure of the geriatric depression scale. *International Psychogeriatrics* 3:23-28.

Sohlberg, M. M., and C. A. Mateer. 1987. Effectiveness of an attention training program. *Journal of Clinical and Experimental Neuropychology* 19:117–130.

Stankov, L. 1988. Aging, intelligence and attention. *Psychology and Aging* 3(2):59-74.

Teasdale, G., and B. Jennett. 1974. Assessment of coma and impairment of consciousness: A practical scale. *Lancet* 2:81-84.

Thurman, D. J., J. E. Sniezek, D. Johnson, A. Greenspan, and S. M. Smith. 1994. *Guidelines for Surveillance of Central Nervous System Injury*. Atlanta: Centers for Disease Control and Prevention.

Tortora, G., and S. Grabowski. 1993. *The Special Senses: Principles of Anatomy and Physiology*. 7th ed. New York: HarperCollins College Publishers.

Yesavage, J. A., T. L. Brink, T. L. Rose, O. Lum, V. Huang, M. B. Adey, and V. O. Leirer. 1983. Development and validation of a geriatric depression screening scale: A preliminary report. *Journal of Psychiatric Research* 17:37-49.

Douglas J. Mason, Psy.D., is a neuropsychologist who specializes in the diagnosis and rehabilitation of people with cognitive dysfunction. He completed his internship at the University of Tennessee in Knoxville, TN, and his residency at Duke University in Durham, NC. He has served on the state of Florida's Brain and Spinal Cord Injury Rehabilitation Counsel. He is the author of *The Memory Workbook* and *The Memory Doctor* (to be released in May 2005). His Web site is **www.memorydr.com.**

Some Other
New Harbinger Titles

A Cancer Patient's Guide to Overcoming Depression and Anxiety, Item 5044 $19.95

The Diabetes Lifestyle Book, Item 5167 $16.95

Solid to the Core, Item 4305 $14.95

Staying Focused in the Age of Distraction, Item 433X $16.95

Living Beyond Your Pain, Item 4097 $19.95

Fibromyalgia & Chronic Fatigue Syndrome, Item 4593 $14.95

Your Miraculous Back, Item 4526 $18.95

TriEnergetics, Item 4453 $15.95

Emotional Fitness for Couples, Item 4399 $14.95

The MS Workbook, Item 3902 $19.95

Depression & Your Thyroid, Item 4062 $15.95

The Eating Wisely for Hormonal Balance Journal, Item 3945 $15.95

Healing Adult Acne, Item 4151 $15.95

The Memory Doctor, Item 3708 $11.95

The Emotional Wellness Way to Cardiac Health, Item 3740 $16.95

The Cyclothymia Workbook, Item 383X $18.95

The Matrix Repatterning Program for Pain Relief, Item 3910 $18.95

Transforming Stress, Item 397X $10.95

Eating Mindfully, Item 3503 $13.95

Living with RSDS, Item 3554 $16.95

The Ten Hidden Barriers to Weight Loss, Item 3244 $11.95

The Sjogren's Syndrome Survival Guide, Item 3562 $15.95

Stop Feeling Tired, Item 3139 $14.95

Responsible Drinking, Item 2949 $19.95

The Mitral Valve Prolapse/Dysautonomia Survival Guide, Item 3031 $14.95

The Vulvodynia Survival Guide, Item 2914 $16.95

The Multifidus Back Pain Solution, Item 2787 $12.95

Move Your Body, Tone Your Mood, Item 2752 $17.95

The Woman's Book of Sleep, Item 2493 $14.95

The Trigger Point Therapy Workbook, second edition, Item 3759 $19.95

Fibromyalgia and Chronic Myofascial Pain Syndrome, 2nd edition, Item 2388 $19.95

Rosacea, Item 2248 $14.95

Coping with Chronic Fatigue Syndrome, Item 0199 $13.95

Call **toll free, 1-800-748-6273,** or log on to our online bookstore at **www.newharbinger.com** to order. Have your Visa or Mastercard number ready. Or send a check for the titles you want to New Harbinger Publications, Inc., 5674 Shattuck Ave., Oakland, CA 94609. Include $4.50 for the first book and 75¢ for each additional book, to cover shipping and handling. (California residents please include appropriate sales tax.) Allow two to five weeks for delivery.

Prices subject to change without notice.